T0303363

Miracle Survivors

Miracle Survivors

Beating the Odds of Incurable Cancer

TAMI BOEHMER

WITH A WORD FROM
BERNIE SIEGEL, MD

AND FOREWORD BY
CURTIS ELLSWORTH SALGADO

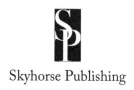

Skyhorse Publishing

Skyhorse Publishing books may be purchased in bulk at special discounts for sales promotion, corporate gifts, fund-raising, or educational purposes. Special editions can also be created to specifications. For details, contact the Special Sales Department, Skyhorse Publishing, 307 West 36th Street, 11th Floor, New York, NY 10018 or info@skyhorsepublishing.com.

Skyhorse® and Skyhorse Publishing® are registered trademarks of Skyhorse Publishing, Inc.®, a Delaware corporation.

Visit our website at www.skyhorsepublishing.com.

10 9 8 7 6 5 4 3 2 1

Library of Congress Cataloging-in-Publication Data is available on file.

Cover design by Jane Sheppard
Cover photo credit Thinkstock

Print ISBN: 978-1-62914-569-3
Ebook ISBN: 978-1-63220-048-8

Printed in the United States of America

Dedication

This book is dedicated to the two most important people in my life: my husband Mike and daughter Chrissy. You have stuck by and supported me through so many ups and downs. I love you dearly and would not be here today to write this book if it weren't for you.

In Memory of

Eleanor Alston, Linda Croucher, Debbi Dempsey, Peter Devereaux, Christine Dittmann, Sally Hawkins, Nevine Latif, Evan Mattingly, Susan Meyers, Pattie Noel, Nancy Oliverias, Lisa Quintana, Vanessa Tiemeier, Ashley Oehler, Buzz Sheffield, Cyndi Wenck, and the many other wonderful individuals with whom I traveled this cancer journey.

And my brother Mitch Greenfield, father Irv Greenfield, stepmother Jean, and my grandmother Shirley Reis—I know you are with me and guiding me every day. I love you and know you would be proud of this work.

Acknowledgements

My deepest gratitude goes to all of the amazing people who shared their stories for this book. You are an inspiration to me and so many others.

I owe so much to my husband Mike Boehmer, who patiently helped proofread each story after long days of work. I also want to thank my agent Cynthia Zigmund, who believed in my vision, gave me excellent direction, and worked diligently to find a publishing home. And to my editor, Marianna Dworak, and the rest of the people at Skyhorse Publishing: Thank you for taking a chance on me and bringing *Miracle Survivors* to fruition.

Thanks to Mary Beth Bauer who quickly and proficiently helped transcribe hours and hours of interviews with no complaint. And to Lori Schulte and Patricia Scriveri who each graciously transcribed a story free of charge.

I wanted to give a shout-out to Beth Franks, who continues to encourage me and offer her sage advice. And last but not least, to my daughter Chrissy, who understood when Mom was on the phone or busily writing when she came from school.

There are so many people in my life who have supported and encouraged me along the way. If I haven't put your names on this page, know that you're always in my heart.

Table of Contents

A Word from Bernie Siegel, MD

Bestselling author of Love, Medicine and Miracles: The Art of Healing, *and dozens of other books.*

Miracle Survivors is a book that everyone should read because it is filled with the wisdom of those who have confronted their mortality and let it become their teacher. When we are willing to ask of ourselves, "What am I to learn from this journey through hell?" we learn to nourish our lives and pay attention to our hunger for living. We use it to guide us and heal our lives. Healing our bodies is a side effect.

Self-induced healing is not an accident or a spontaneous lucky occurrence. It takes work, and the work is learning to love ourselves, our lives, and our bodies. When we do that, our bodies do the best they can to keep us alive.

As you read the stories shared here pay attention to the common themes because they are the lessons to be learned from survivors and the survivor personality.

I've learned much as a physician who has counseled cancer patients for many decades. In all of my books, which feature inspiring lessons from people either living with or healed of cancer, I reflect upon what each story teaches us about not just surviving, but thriving. My latest book, *The Art of Healing*, demonstrates how our unconscious can both communicate with and assist us in healing through dreams and drawings.

Tami Boehmer allows the stories to speak for themselves. Because of the simple way each person presents how they're living the message, it can be easy for some readers to miss the wisdom it contains. In other words, tourists are often not aware of what is obvious to the natives. So please read the stories slowly and thoughtfully, paying special attention to each Lessons Learned section. And make sure to refer to "The

Common Attributes of Miracle Survivors" addressed at the beginning of this book. These commonalities, coupled with the stories, speak volumes of their effectiveness.

Miracle Survivors is not just for people who are threatened with illness; it's for everyone who wants to live a longer, healthier, and happier life. Remember that life is uncertain, so do what makes you happy and eat dessert first. When you live, your chocolate ice cream miracles and self-healing do occur.

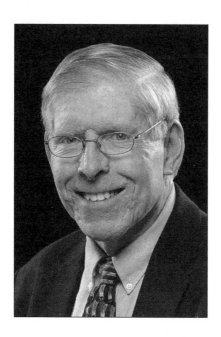

Introduction

Dave deBronkart, (AKA e-Patient Dave)
Nashua, NH
Age 64
Diagnosed in 2007 with stage IV renal cancer

Hope is a resource—a real, scientifically verified resource.

Jerome Groopman MD's excellent book, *The Anatomy of Hope: How People Prevail in the Face of Illness*, cites evidence from well-controlled experiments demonstrating that when challenged, patients' bodies will perform differently based on their minds' expectation. We're not just talking about their experience of pain—scientists measured a substantial difference in their physiological response, comparable in strength to a drug. Dr. Groopman calls hope "a catalyst in the crucible of cure," and concludes, "There is an authentic biology of hope."

He writes, "Hope, unlike optimism, is rooted in unalloyed reality. . . . Hope acknowledges the significant obstacles and deep pitfalls along the path. True hope has no room for delusion. . . . Clear-eyed, hope gives us the courage to confront our circumstances and the capacity to surmount them," he continues. "For all my patients, hope, true hope, has proved as important as any medication."

When you believe there's no hope, your biology shifts. It's as if your system gives up. Until you decide it's your time to go, don't give up hope. You have no idea what might happen.

I wasn't optimistic when I was diagnosed with stage IV kidney cancer. I vividly pictured my mother's face as she buried me. But I was persistent. You could say one of my mottos in life is, "There's got to be a way to figure this out. And if it doesn't work, you try something else. And if that doesn't work, you try another option."

I asked my oncologist Dr. McDermott—one of the best scientists in the world for this disease—about my prognosis, and he wisely didn't give me any specific number. But I wanted to know (I have a big appetite for information) so I did some digging online, and eventually figured out that my median survival was twenty-four weeks after diagnosis. Every article I read about the disease said, "Outlook is bleak." "Prognosis is grim." "Almost all patients are incurable."

Considering how many tumors I had throughout my body, the prognosis wasn't surprising. But on the other hand, that data was about a decade old, so it didn't reflect current success rates. (My patient community knows that all five-year survival data is at least five years out of date!)

I presented my situation to my patient community on the Association of Cancer Online Resources (ACOR). One of the first things people said to me was, "Well, if you don't want to die of kidney cancer, here's what you do—live long enough to die of something else first." I know a guy whose trick is living long enough for another treatment to be developed—he's done it several times already. Hearing these things helped me feel like maybe I wasn't doomed and gave me plenty of good reasons not give up hope.

They steered me to a famous article by a scientist named Stephen Jay Gould, called "The Median Isn't the Message." Gould described his experience after he was diagnosed with mesothelioma and explained why median survival estimates are useless: They're useful to the scientists who use them to compare things, but not useful for predicting the outcome of any individual.

Here's how the median works: Let's say researchers follow a group of twenty-five people. When the thirteenth patient (the middle person of the twenty-five) dies, that's the median—they can publish their paper, with a median survival time. But they can't publish information on the other half of the population—because they don't know how long they'll live: at publication, those people haven't died yet!

So it's important to view median survival figures in context. Many clinicians, including good ones, have forgotten that. They were trained to look at what the literature says. But it's a scientific mistake for a doctor or a nurse to look at a median and say, "You've got about six months to live."

Groopman also talks about his medical training and how he was taught not to give patients false hope. I can imagine it's a tragic thing if you try to give somebody encouragement and they come back a year later and say, "But doctor, you told me I would survive."

But there are ways to handle this, accurately and truthfully. I remember a doctor who told me how he used to reply, "Probably not," when a patient would ask, "Can you save me?" He saw the life go out of them. Now he says, "I don't know—but we'll try." We all want to hear doctors tell us they're going to do everything they can to beat this. But we also need information that will help us do this.

I was in a clinical trial using the drug interleukin, and I knew that the side effects could be severe enough to kill a patient. My doctors didn't have any literature on the subject, so I thought, Where is the patient tutorial on how to deal with side effects? And you know what? It didn't exist. I didn't find a word about it on any scientific website.

Many clinicians have been taught there's no reason to worry a patient about something like severe side effects because it might not happen to them. Why burden them with that knowledge, right? To me, that is extremely paternalistic. The assumption sometimes is patients can't handle the information; it's too much for them. The underlying view is that the patient isn't a capable partner in attacking the problem.

So I turned to my patient community and received seventeen first-hand stories of people who have been through interleukin treatments. When the side effects hit me, I knew what was happening and I knew what other people had done to alleviate the symptoms.

I also received a lot of wisdom and support regarding the importance of attitude. Throughout treatment, I had a big metastasis in the femur. If you think having side effects like nausea and diarrhea are fun, imagine having them when you can't move fast because your leg is breaking and you're using a walker. But I said, "You know what? Option one is I just die, and I don't have to worry about diarrhea. Option two is I'm alive and I have to worry about diarrhea."

At one point, I had capillary leak syndrome, where the walls of your capillaries open and essentially all fluid runs out. Eventually you have no blood pressure, which is a nifty way to die. My legs blew up like water balloons and my blood pressure dropped to 50/30, so they had to discontinue my treatment. There were times when to fall asleep, I had to literally say to myself, "Good night cancer. You'll be there in the morning," so I could just stop thinking about it.

Clinicians are taught to understand the biology of the disease, what causes it, and what to do about it. But it's very different from living with the disease and managing your life. The Institute of Medicine's report, "Best Care at Lower Cost: The Path to Continuously Learning Health Care in America," made an important point: Medicine needs to be "anchored" (that's the word they used) on the patient's point of view. It lists patient/clinician partnerships as one of four elements essential to the future of medicine.

If the patient's perspective is essential to the future of medicine, you as the the patient need to express your point of view. The core of empowerment is to be conscious of what you want and to express it. You can't fault another person for not responding to a wish you haven't expressed. Patient empowerment isn't about demanding information from your doctors, it's about expressing yourself in a respectful manner. You can say, "I like to understand as much as I can. Can I ask some questions?" If the answer to that is, "No, I'll tell you what you need to know," then you might want to find a different doctor.

My oncologist recognized the value of this. He agreed to be quoted in an essay I recently wrote for the *British Medical Journal,* saying, "I don't know if you could have tolerated enough medicine to survive if you hadn't been so informed and prepared."

I want people to know about their options and possibilities. To me it's a shame if somebody never finds out that something was possible or finds out too late. I learned that three out of four metastatic kidney cancer patients never hear that interleukin exists as a treatment option. All the information about interleukin on guidelines doctors follow, last I heard, is ten years out of date.

There are plenty of reasons to think for yourself and find out if there are treatments that other people don't know about. In my case, my treatment was a clinical trial of a new protocol. Interleukin had been approved by the FDA in the 1990s, but my trial was studying a new way to administer it. According to the hypothesis in the trial, my type of tumor should not have responded. But it did.

Almost all the conversation about changing medicine is about its problems, gaps, and shortfalls. But the reality is I'm here because medicine saved my ass. In the March 2013 issue of *General Surgery News,* Jon White, MD, wrote that more than half of all the humans who have ever reached the age sixty-five are alive today. That becomes credible when you consider that at the end of World War II, there were 2.3 billion humans. Today, there are more than three times as many people and a lot more of them are living to be older.

This makes a good case for being an engaged patient. Medicine has succeeded in many ways. They're predicting in the future that more and more of us are going to live to be over seventy or eighty. Either we will crush the system with a huge influx of patients or we're going to be doing more to take care of ourselves.

It's great to be alive. It's wonderful to be around to witness wonderful moments like the birth of my granddaughter Zoe. It was great to be part of my daughter Lindsey's wedding and that she didn't have to say, "I wish Dad could have been here."

I wasn't sure I would be able to witness these events, but there were others who carried hope for me. When I was first diagnosed, my best friend Dorron Levy, a rigorous and deep-thinking scientist from Israel, came with his family to visit for a long weekend. His brother, a leading physician in Israel, had read my data on my patient portal and told him I was basically screwed.

It was costly for them: four short-notice plane tickets, hotel and all. And since at the time I still had the financial stress of owning two houses (I had just moved back to the Boston area from Minnesota), they insisted on buying all our meals.

Years later I said to him, "You must have felt you were coming to say goodbye." He replied, "Nothing could be farther from the truth. I was certain you would make it. We came to give you hope."

Hearing this from a "high priest of evidence" made my jaw drop. He said, "Dave, in physics right now there are two contending factions—reductionism and emergence. Reductionists want to eliminate all confounding variables to get repeatable results. Emergence is the study of what tiny influences lead to new patterns as the chaos unfolds." His action in "giving hope" was an injection into the chaos.

Think about this as you read the following stories, which are presented to give you hope. Whether it's belief-based or a scientific hypothesis, hope is vital. Let it be a spark, igniting you to become a more-informed, engaged patient and encourage others to do the same.

Dave deBronkart, known on the Internet as e-Patient Dave, is the author of the highly rated Let Patients Help: A Patient Engagement Handbook *and one of the world's leading advocates for patient engagement. A blogger, health policy advisor, and international keynote speaker, he is today the best-known spokesman for the patient engagement movement.*

A co-founder and current co-chair of the Society for Participatory Medicine, e-Patient Dave has appeared in Time, US News, USA Today, Wired, MIT Technology Review, *and* HealthLeaders, *among other publications and medical journals. His compelling TEDx Talk "Let Patients Help" was for years in the top half of most-watched TED talks of all time with subtitles in twenty-six languages. For more information, visit* www.epatientdave.com.

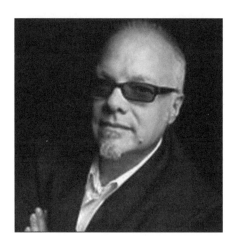

Foreword

CURTIS ELLSWORTH SALGADO
Portland, OR
60 years old
Diagnosed in 2007 with stage IV liver cancer

This book is important because people need to have hope. You need it to fight the good fight. It's not all doom and gloom. The heavy thing about cancer is you know the way you'll probably die, but it doesn't mean you're going to die of cancer. You don't know; you can't predict it. But I think you need that positive reinforcement because it will change the way your body responds. I believe you can change outcomes.

People gave me a lot of love and prayers when I was diagnosed with liver cancer. I must have heard about eighty times, "My entire church prayed for you." That was a lot of prayer.

I grew up in a family that was very open-minded, loving, and blessed. They weren't into church or any kind of religion. If my mother wanted to go to church, it was probably because she didn't have a babysitter and needed a nap. I'm not Christian or Muslim, but I believe in the power of prayer and positive thinking. I think this book is like a prayer itself.

When I was kid, though, religion was a sticking point. I was shunned by my friends in the sixth grade. For some reason, they turned on me. Kids were very mean to me, pushed books out of my hands, and wouldn't talk to me. I found out later it was because my mother had a party with neighborhood mothers, and she revealed we didn't go to church. My parents might have believed in God and a higher power, but didn't belong to a denomination. The parents went home and told their kids to stay away from Curtis.

Music turned everything around. My father bought me a Fender Mustang guitar and Princeton amp when I was in seventh grade. Someone found out I was playing guitar, and the two most popular kids in my grade came up to me and said, "Hey man, let's go over to my house and play." After that, I was in a new clique and was never bothered again.

Music has always been a part of my life. My folks were jazz enthusiasts. They loved swing music like Count Basie, Benny Goodman, and Anita O'Day. My father loved cats like Fats Waller, Louis Armstrong, and Ray Charles. He had all the 78s, which I still keep.

I've been singing ever since kindergarten. My teacher pinned a note to my chest and said, "Take this to your mom." I brought it home to my mom and she said, "Oh, your teacher says you have a nice voice and you're to learn these songs." My mother could play piano and could read music quite well, so we rehearsed. I learned the songs and sang in front of an audience at a school assembly.

That night, as I was standing on stage with a partner, singing "I've Been Working on the Railroad," the guy froze. I elbowed him and said, "Come on, sing," but he clammed up, so I belted it out. The audience was laughing and I was thinking, Wow, they're digging on me! And I was hooked from that moment on.

When I was thirteen, I met an older kid and I started experimenting with drinking and drugs. It wasn't every day, but it was something that occupied my time. I remember when I was fifteen and at a party with older kids; a guy stuck headphones on me and shot me up with a speed ball (a mixture of heroin and coke). It was a rush, and it was fun. We didn't know any better or the damage it would do in the future.

I used drugs and drank until I was thirty-five years old. I knew I needed to quit and put myself in treatment. I wasn't having fun anymore, and I overdosed a couple of times. I knew I was going to kill myself, and I liked me better than that. I now have twenty-five years of sobriety under my belt.

When I quit drugs in 1988, I found out I had Hepatitis C and moderate cirrhosis of the liver. I went to a doctor, who told me about a medicine called interferon, but it only had a 30 percent recovery rate, and the side effects were wicked. I had to inject it three days of every week for a year and feel like crap, so I rejected it.

In 2006, I wasn't working much and didn't have a record out to promote, so I thought I better start checking on myself. I was starting to hurt and wondered how much damage the Hepatitis had done. Tests showed I had only 20 percent liver function, no platelets, and an inflamed pancreas. I felt it was time to get interferon, which was being used with another drug Ribavirin to heal Hepatitis. I was a good candidate for the drug cocktail, but I had no health insurance.

I had changed insurance companies because mine was charging more than six hundred dollars a month. When I went to another insurance company for a lower rate, the representative suggested not including my Hepatitis diagnosis in the application. A week later, he retired and I learned he was building up his quota beforehand. When I tried to get the interferon, they called me up and said, "You lied on your insurance application, so we are going to take you off the program."

A close friend, who was good at working with hospital administration, convinced them to give me a payment plan, so I could get the $17,000 treatment for a low out-of-pocket amount.

Two weeks later, I was having breakfast at a restaurant and experienced pain that nearly knocked me to my knees. I called my friend again and told her I was having a gallstone attack. We went to her house and I kicked back, waiting for it to go away. Meanwhile she called the gastroenterologist who told her to take me to the emergency room. I said, "I'm not going to the ER; do you know how expensive it is to go there?" About four hours later, I said, "Get me to the emergency room; it's not going away."

When we were in the ER, they gave me something for pain. I felt great and said, "I'm going home." They interrupted me and said, "You are going to get in the hospital. Your gallbladder is shot; it's red and infected. You need surgery to have it removed. By law, insurance or not, they have to take you." All I could think about was, "I can't afford this!"

Because I had no platelets, which coagulates blood, they had to wait to do surgery. My surgeon, Dr. Hanson, saw a spot on my CT scan, and performed a biopsy. The next morning, I decided to leave the hospital. I had been there four days and still didn't have my gallbladder removed and nobody was telling me anything. It was costing me too much, so I went home to my friend's house.

The next morning, Dr. Hanson called to tell me they didn't get enough information from the biopsy, and I had to come in to get another one. I said, "Why did they miss the spot?" He replied, "Spot? What are you talking about? You have a tumor as big as a lemon, and I think it's cancer."

I just sat down on the floor and screamed "F***!" as loud as I could. I didn't think about it; it's just what happened.

I still think about it every day. On March 21, my friend, my manager, and I went to Dr. Hanson's office and learned I had a five-and-a-half-centimeter tumor. I needed a liver transplant. Because of its size, however, I couldn't get one. They wouldn't risk a transplant on a tumor bigger than five centimeters.

I said, "Are you telling me I'm going to die?" He started to say something, and I put up my hand and said, "Stop! What would you do if you were me?" He suggested checking out transplant centers and getting on a waiting list, but he didn't think most of them would take me. He told us I only had six to seven months before my tumor spread. At that point, I couldn't get a liver transplant, and I would probably die of liver cancer.

Every day I was tested, but I didn't give up. And I had so many amazing people that helped. Andrea Crawford, my ex-girlfriend, stepped back into my life. She gave up a six-figure job, moved into her garage, and rented her house. Andrea studied a medical dictionary to understand the jargon and started researching places in the US where there was less competition for a liver transplant. Doctors told us it took nine months to two years to get on a waiting list.

Andrea said, "I'm the same blood type as you; I can donate part of my liver!" I answered, "You can't give me your liver; you're my ex-girlfriend. I'm not going to take your liver." She told me to get over it and that it would be too late by the time they found a liver for me.

Without insurance, we estimated it would cost $800,000 to $1 million for transplant surgery, medications, and anti-rejection drugs, as well as twenty-four-hour after care for at least the first four weeks after surgery.

I'm blessed to have some famous friends. Bonnie Raitt paid three months of my rent. My manager, Shane Tappindeorf, put together a benefit concert for me at the Rose Garden, a huge coliseum which the city of Portland donated to us. The show featured Steve Miller, Robert Cray Band, Taj Mahal, Phantom Blues Band, Everclear, and Little Charlie and the Nightcats, plus my band. We made over $200,000.

We were at the seven-month point when we were ready to do the transplant. Miraculously, they discovered Andrea's liver was abnormally large for a girl her size, so it was a perfect contender. But they also discovered my heart was beating irregularly and they were afraid I'd die on the table. We needed to wait three weeks. I said, "Three weeks! This is month seven. I'm supposed to have six maybe seven months before this spreads!"

My doctor gave me blood pressure medicine. About a week and half later, they called to tell me my heart was doing better, so they could do the operation. But here's the glitch: Their financial department told us we were $100,000 short, and they weren't going to perform the operation until I paid for it. I thought, Where in God's name am I going to get $100,000? Unbelievably, two friends at the last minute gave me their life savings to cover the costs.

We were good to go for the operation. The head honcho of the transplant department said, "We decided to put you on the donor list just for the hell of it." I said, "Why would you do that? The operation is in five days and it will take me another nine months to get accepted." He answered, "Well who knows? Maybe something will happen."

Three days later while we were waiting to do the operation with Andrea, the doctor called and said, "Take a shower, put on your pj's, and come down. We think we have a liver for you." What are the odds of that?

I got to the hospital at 6 a.m. They rolled me into the operating room, and there was a team of surgeons waiting for me. I played with Santana for a brief period of my career and they obviously knew about it. "Oye Como Va" was playing on a huge boom box, and the surgical team was dancing and sticking their thumbs in the air at me. And just then, the mask came down.

I knew I could die on the table because there was a risk of a stroke, or I'd wake up and find out I didn't get the transplant because they found cancer. People don't realize that liver transplants are the Super Bowl of transplants.

I woke up with a tube down my throat, one in my nose, and tubes running out of my arms. My sister Wendy, who was there with Andrea, handed me a piece of paper because I couldn't talk. I was kind of delirious and drugged up and wrote, "That was wonderful; I can't wait to do it again."

A few weeks later the surgeon came to my hospital room and said, "We have found a microscopic invasion in a small, insignificant blood vessel in your liver. We still have your old liver and we've gone over it with a fine-toothed comb. It's so small and so fresh that we don't know if it's a metastasis."

I asked, "Does that mean a cancer cell could jump into the blood vessel and take the subway out to parts unknown?" She said there was a

50/50 chance that could happen, and then told me they wouldn't have done the transplant had they known about it.

I received scans every four months. At eight months, they found a tiny spot in my lung. They weren't sure it was cancer, but they wanted to take it out right away no matter what it was. I had a really important gig to do, so I said to wait another three months and see if it grew.

When the time came, they took out the tumor, which had grown to the size of a marble. Sure enough it was liver cancer that had metastasized to the lung.

After surgery, a cancer specialist came in my room and asked, "Where are the others? You only have one tumor, and you're immune-suppressed because of the anti-rejection medications. You should have about four or five. I don't know why it happens, and we can't explain it, but you're very lucky. You're a miracle."

She stood up to leave and I said, "Wait, wait! I have questions!" She just said, "Good luck Mr. Salgado," and left.

If you can survive for five years with this particular kind of cancer, they say you're pretty much good to go. The summer of 2012, I went in for my five-year checkup. The doctor told me, "I hate to say it, but we see something." It was liver cancer and back in the same place.

Cancer changed everything for me. As a musician and entertainer, my dream was to fill up coliseums and rock the world. But now it just doesn't matter. I'm extremely blessed and lucky. I have nothing to complain about. I'm already rich and famous . . . rich in friends and famous in the eyes of God.

Every six months, I go to my doctor at Providence Medical Center. He's either going to say everything is okay or change my whole life by saying he sees something. It's high anxiety. If he comes in and he's not holding an envelope or slides, I say, "Oh God, thank you!" Last time he said, "Everything is good, buddy."

Cancer brings you to the very zenith of humanity. It's very emotionally deep. It makes you think of your place on the planet and what you've accomplished. This is the point where you realize life is finite and every day is a gift.

Don't give up. Look at me; I had all sorts of obstacles. I had no health insurance and couldn't afford my care; and now it's all paid off. It's just one of the miracles I experienced.

It's truly about being in the moment. You can't trip about the past or flip out about the future. I don't dwell on the negative. I always say I had cancer, not have. I feel very strongly that everything is gonna be alright.

Photo by Paul Natkin/Photo Reserve courtesy of Alligator Records.

Curtis Salgado is an award-winning vocalist and harmonica player who tours the world with his band to venues ranging from the Chicago Blues Festival to Poland's Blues Alive Festival. He has shared the stage with music greats, such as Robert Cray, Steve Miller, Carlos Santana, Muddy Waters, and Bonnie Raitt. Curtis, who befriended John Belushi in the late 70s, was the inspiration for The Blues Brothers. As a nod to Salgado, Cab Calloway's character in the film was named Curtis. For more information, visit **www.curtissalgado.com.**

The Common Attributes of "Miracle Survivors"

When I started interviewing individuals for my first book, *From Incurable to Incredible*, I had only seven months under my belt as a stage IV breast cancer survivor. My primary goal was to inspire hope and show that it was possible to beat the odds of a terminal or incurable prognosis.

As I was compiling stories, I noticed many similarities among the featured survivors. *Miracle Survivors* introduces new stories, but I found the same common characteristics applied as those in my previous book.

While I call the individuals in this book "miracle survivors," overcoming the odds wasn't something that just happened to them. Each person took a very active role in overcoming their challenges, whether it was activating their faith or transforming their lifestyle. Rather than passively accepting their circumstances, they decided to transform them by:

- Being proactive participants in their health care.
- Refusing to buy into statistics and the death sentences many of them were given.
- Never giving up, no matter what. They may have had down times, but were able to pull themselves together and do what they needed to do.
- Relying on support from family, loved ones, or support groups. These connections gave them a reason to carry on.
- Choosing to look on the bright side and see the gifts cancer brings.
- Giving back and making a difference in other people's lives, whether it was fundraising, lobbying, or supporting other survivors.

- Having a strong sense of faith. Even if they didn't believe in God, they believed in something larger than themselves.
- Viewing their lives as transformed by their experience.

I share this with one caveat. Cancer is tricky, and I've had many dear friends who have passed away who had these qualities. Did they live longer than they would have? I don't know. Did they live better because they did these things? I'd have to say yes. Their passing does not make them any less miraculous. They made the world a better place for me and so many others.

There are no winners or losers or the right or wrong way to deal with cancer and other major life challenges. But I know from experience and from talking with hundreds of people living with cancer that how we live our life is a choice. The people in the following stories choose to live with love, hope, and compassion. If you see yourself in their journeys or are inspired to follow their examples, then my job is done.

Hugs, hope, and healing!
Tami Boehmer

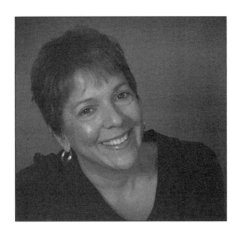

My Story

My survival instinct was strongly activated early in childhood. Born to parents that, despite best intentions, were incapable of caring for me, I was left with my grandmother at the tender age of three. My parents and two older brothers, Mitch and Doug, moved to Philadelphia, hundreds of miles away. I returned to my family at age seven, but it was a bumpy ride to say the least. My family was fraught with drug addiction and mental illness. I learned to adapt as best as I could and became a little adult trying to fix my family's problems.

As an adult, I went to psychologists and twelve-step programs to heal my past. After working my way through college, I began a profession in public relations in the health care field. It eventually appeared to be an ironic choice. In April 2002, I gained first-hand experience of the health care system after being diagnosed with stage II, estrogen/progesterone-positive breast cancer.

I was four days shy of my thirty-ninth birthday, and had been married five years. My daughter, Chrissy, was just three years old. I remember my breast surgeon calling our home at 10 p.m. to deliver the news. My husband Mike literally collapsed on the floor. I went into shock and switched to professional mode, taking down notes and gathering information.

I had no family history, which I later learned was common. I led a mostly healthy lifestyle, I thought. It was just a terrible twist of fate. I did the standard chemo regime at the time: a combination of Adriamycin (AKA, the Red Devil), Cytoxan, and 5FU, lumpectomy and radiation, followed by five years of taking the drug Tamoxifen. My oncologist told me my prognosis was excellent.

Being a worrier all my life, I still had anxiety about the cancer returning, and worse, that I would eventually die from this disease. I felt powerless that I could do anything to impact the situation. I went to too many funerals of younger friends who had breast cancers from my support group.

I became stressed out after being laid off from a job I loved, and then quickly started at a new job that was very unhealthy. I lost sleep and serenity, and my family was impacted as well. It seemed that I worried more about a gap in my resume than taking care of me and my family.

It all came to a head in February 2008. I insisted on seeing my breast surgeon a month earlier than my regular checkup because of a large lump I discovered in my right armpit. I had worried from time to time about some swelling and hardness. Since the swelling would go down, my surgeon thought it was probably hormonal. I was so relieved, I didn't question it. But a month or two later, the swelling didn't go away, and I started experiencing extreme pain in my arm.

Now I wanted answers. She sat me down with the results of the ultrasound, and gave me one of the saddest looks you could imagine. My worst nightmare came true—after five years of being cancer-free, it had come back with a vengeance. The tumor was a very large nine centimeters in diameter.

The next step was a barrage of scans to see if the cancer spread. I was working at a large teaching hospital, so I could easily slip downstairs to the radiology department. I remember retrieving my results and sitting in my office, staring at my PET scan report. There were spots in lymph nodes in my chest and, most worrisome, my liver. It was stage IV breast cancer. There was no one else around, so I let myself fall apart. In a few hours, my husband and I were sitting in my oncologist's office wondering how this could happen.

We decided to go to an oncologist at a very prestigious institution two thousand miles away for a second opinion. We were expecting hope, maybe a clinical trial recommendation. Instead, she told me, "You could live two years or twenty years, but you will die of breast cancer."

My husband squeezed my hand as we both started to cry. I knew my prognosis wasn't great, but hearing those words was devastating. What about my daughter Chrissy? She was only in third grade, and she needed me. It all seemed so unreal. Then this little seed of strength emerged as I responded, "I'm too stubborn to die."

When we were in the car, my grief turned into anger. "How does she know how long I have to live?" I said. "She doesn't even know me!" At that moment, I affirmed I was going to prove her wrong.

I remembered reading a line in Bernie Siegel's wonderful book, *Love, Medicine and Miracles*. He talked about how his patients who did best were not the "good patients," who smiled and acquiesced to everything. The "exceptional cancer patients," as he called them, were the complainers who asked good questions—the ones who, frankly, were pains in the ass. They were the ones who made it despite a terrible prognosis.

These patients, Bernie describes, are "self-reliant and seek solutions rather than slip into depression. They interpret problems as redirections."

I knew I needed more than medical treatment to get well. I had always gained strength from other cancer survivors who had overcome the disease to lead flourishing lives. Faced with a dire diagnosis, I needed to talk with other metastatic cancer survivors who beat the odds. And I was determined to find out how they did it so I could do it myself.

I thought of Buzz Sheffield,* a volunteer prayer chaplain at our church. Buzz was always up in the front row with a snazzy suit and dazzling smile. You could almost see the light of God emanating from him.

In one of those "coincidences," a few months earlier, I saw Buzz sitting in the courtyard of the hospital where I worked. It was a beautiful sunny day, and Buzz looked peaceful as he read a book. As usual, I was in a hurry, dashing to meet a TV reporter who was doing a story on one of our patients.

He told me he was waiting for tests, and previous ones showed he had cancer all over his body. I stood there in shock. I would have never guessed that this active, robust man had anything wrong with him. We didn't know each other well at the time, but I felt a special connection with him from that moment on.

After church that Sunday, I asked him about his tests and illness. He told me he had carcinoid cancer, a rare, slow-moving disease that often attacks the intestines and other parts of the body where hormones are produced. Four years earlier, doctors told him he had three to six months to live. His cancer was so extensive, chemotherapy wasn't an option. But he refused to listen to their doomsday predictions and chose to focus on healing. To look at him and his active lifestyle, I knew whatever he was doing was working.

The first night after getting my dreaded diagnosis, I needed to talk to someone who understood what I was going through, and most important, was doing well. I gave Buzz a call.

He told me to not give up, stay in the moment, and remain positive. Buzz talked about his strong spiritual connection, healthy diet, and exercise routine. I met more teachers along the way and started following their recommendations as I went through surgery and chemotherapy treatments.

I made some significant changes in my lifestyle. I left my stressful job and started a daily routine of exercise, prayer, visualization, and affirmations. While I was waiting in the car to pick up my daughter from school or in line at the store, I would visualize my immune system melting the cancer cells away. As I drank water—and lots of it—I would see myself cleansing the residue of dead cancer cells out of my body. While taking a shower, I talked to my body, urging it to clear out the cancer and thanking it for its amazing work.

To learn how I could build my immune system, I consulted with a holistic physician and read books on holistic healing. I spent time purchasing organic produce and supplements with cancer-fighting properties. I even gave up sugar, which I loved, with the exception of really dark chocolate. I started using eco-friendly cleaners and natural shampoos and lotions.

I focused on serving others in my breast cancer support group, at church, and by delivering meals to elderly people in my neighborhood. Most of all, I began to devote time to enriching all of my relationships, especially with my family, myself, and God.

All of these practices gave me a sense of power, because I knew I was doing something concrete to support my healing. And it seemed to be working. Remarkably, my side effects were minimal and my tumors shrank with every scan.

But still, I fought off depression and was haunted by the sinking feeling I was going to die. With all the focus on myself and getting well, I felt useless and empty. I was searching for meaning in my life.

Mike encouraged me to write a book about my experience, but I thought I was too early in the process to share anything meaningful. That summer, we went on vacation with Mike's family to a beautiful lake in Canada. On one of my daily morning walks, an idea popped into my head. "Why not write a book about other advanced-stage cancer patients and how they beat the odds?" I thought it would be therapeutic for me, and more important, help others. I soon began interviewing cancer survivors from around the country for my first book, *From Incurable to Incredible.*

My cancer has come and gone several times. I have since had a hysterectomy, eight different chemotherapies, biopsies, and a targeted radiation procedure called Selective Internal Radiation Therapy (SIRT), which eliminated the liver tumor.

I actually learned about SIRT from Nancy Hamm, one of the people featured in my first book. Nancy had the procedure, which involves injecting Yttrium 90 (SIR) microspheres into the femoral artery, directly to the liver tumor. Both of my oncologists, one who is considered the top in his profession, discouraged me from getting it. I listened to my research and my gut and had it done. It worked. Four years later, I still have no evidence of disease in my liver.

I'm constantly researching different treatments, seeking second and third opinions, and networking with other survivors. I make sure to have both a consulting, out-of-town oncologist and a local oncologist and come to my visits with lists of questions and ideas. When I make decisions about treatments, I combine information with the feeling in my gut that tells me, "This is the right one."

As I write this, I've been on a fairly new, targeted treatment for estrogen/progesterone-positive breast cancer—Afinitor, along with Aromasin—for more than a year. My first three scans showed regression, and my recent scan was stable, which for someone living with metastatic cancer is very good news.

For me, cancer was a wakeup call. If I didn't learn the first time around, this second bout with cancer certainly caught my attention. Cancer has brought many blessings that I would not have realized without this daunting challenge. Writing this book and my last one is certainly one of them. The process of interviewing the amazing individuals featured in the book and writing their stories has been extremely therapeutic to me. I include their stories, along with ways to heal the body, mind, and spirit, in my blog called "Miracle Survivors."

I shy away from news reports and studies that talk about poor survival rates. Statistics are just numbers that lump together a large, diverse group of individuals. They don't apply to me, and they certainly don't apply to the people I've interviewed for my books and blog.

I've heard so many powerful success stories; it seems beating the odds of terminal cancer is more of a norm, rather than an exception. When I struggle, I think of how the people who shared their stories in my books and on my blog never gave up despite setbacks. And almost all of them are thriving today. It gives me hope and purpose, knowing I'm helping others get through their struggles, too. When I'm feeling down, I know that's when I need to reach out to others. Giving back by mentoring and supporting other cancer survivors helps shorten my pity parties.

But my biggest source of strength, in addition to God, is Mike and Chrissy, who is now fifteen years old. We are a unified team in every way. Mike encourages me to take care of my health—body, mind, and spirit. He's my biggest promoter and staunch supporter. He's there when I cry and get angry and when I celebrate success.

It hasn't been easy, but I've learned to be one of those pain-in-the-ass patients. I'm nice about it, don't get me wrong. But I know that no one has as big of an investment in keeping me alive and well as me. I may not hold a medical degree, but I've learned a lot about breast cancer throughout my twelve-year journey. And I know my body.

If you lead a corporation, you hire good people with expertise to do their jobs. But you're still the boss. That's how I try to look at my medical experience. I have the right to hire and fire doctors. If a doctor gives up and acts like he/she doesn't care, they're off my payroll. I will look for someone who won't give up on me and has new ideas. And I won't just listen to them and follow blindly. I'll do the research myself, consult with other people, and make an educated decision. The buck stops here, as they say.

I constantly visualize being there for Chrissy as she graduates from high school and college. I can almost smell the bouquet as Mike and I walk her down the aisle on her wedding day. That's my goal, and I'm determined to meet it. Over time, I have built my faith that God will fulfill my heart's desire if I continue to work towards it. God did not bring me this far to let me down.

In the meantime, I'm focusing on my wonderful life and living in the moment. Cancer may have been a turning point, but it does not define me. My days are full, and I'm finally giving myself permission to enjoy each and every one of them. I'm no longer just surviving like I was during my turbulent childhood; I'm thriving.

Lessons Learned

- Statistics are just numbers; don't let them define the length of your life.
- Be an informed participant in your health care. Don't be intimidated by your doctor's knowledge. Research, get other opinions, talk to fellow survivors, and ask questions.
- Be sure to take care of your body, mind, and spirit with a clean diet and exercise, and by seeking solace in faith, nature, or whatever you believe is a power greater than yourself.
- Live one day at a time as much as you can. No one can predict the future, so focus on what's good and living life fully.

As I write this, I have learned that Buzz passed away a few days ago. He lived ten years after doctors gave him three to six months to live—a life full of service and joy. Whenever I or anyone else asked Buzz how he was doing, he'd always reply, "Always my best." I believe he is now at his best, free from pain and guiding us from above. For more information about Tami, visit www.miraclesurvivors.com.

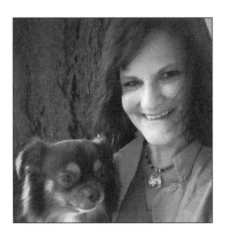

Turning Triple-Negative Into a Positive

BRENDA BEGUIN
Olympia, WA
Age 50
Living with stage IV triple-negative breast cancer since 2010

My experience with cancer came at a young age. When I was fourteen, my aunt was diagnosed with ovarian cancer, so I was tested for the BRCA gene mutation that indicates if you're at high risk for ovarian and breast cancer. I tested positive for the gene.

In 2005, when I was forty-two years old, I was diagnosed with stage III breast cancer. Tests came back that it was triple negative, which means it doesn't respond to estrogen/progesterone receptor- and HER2/neu-targeted therapies. Because of this, it's one of the most aggressive cancers.

It was a stressful time. I got divorced from my first husband and was working while going to school to get certified in billing, coding, and management.

Doctors didn't know back then how serious it was; they just wanted to stick me with a whole bunch of chemotherapy. I was trying to support myself, and I couldn't afford chemo and radiation and paying for my home.

If that wasn't bad enough, when I started radiation, my ex-husband went to court and petitioned to get custody of our daughter. First, he said I didn't have cancer, so I had to go to court proving that I did by providing a doctor's note and records. Once I proved I had cancer, he said I wasn't fit to take care of her because of cancer. Then I had to prove I could still take care of my daughter.

It was extremely traumatic not having a spouse to support me when I needed him. My mom had to fly from Arizona to help me pack my bags because he got custody of my daughter. That meant they could live in our home, so I had to move out and find an apartment. My daughter realized a few months later what her dad had done.

Because of everything he was putting me through, I chose a lumpectomy and opted out of chemo. I just couldn't handle any more. But I got through it and went into remission. I continued with my life, met someone new, and remarried in 2006.

In 2010, I was working in a radiologist's office. We were having some remodeling done in our parking lot, and the building I was working in would shake every time they would dig. I have asthma but didn't usually have a lot of problems . . . until that all started. I got sick with bronchitis and had to wear a mask at work because of the particles that were falling from the ceiling. I brought in a note from my doctor's office that said I shouldn't be sitting in the building while work was going on, but they needed me to work.

I wasn't getting better even though construction was starting to slow down. So I went to my oncologist and told her something wasn't right. My calcium level was really high, and she said they were going to monitor it. I said that it had been a while since I had had a PET scan and she replied, "We're not going to scan you unless you're symptomatic," and that they'd monitor me.

So I went to my family physician and asked for a PET scan, and he said sure and ordered it. When I went to go pick up my report, it said I had what they thought was an enlarged nodule in the right lung.

I remember trying not to panic, but there was a sense of urgency. I was disgusted that there was something in my body I didn't know should be there or not. Of course, working in the radiology office, I went right away to the doctors who I worked with. It's like a family; they took really good care of me, and we started doing testing.

The nodule was so small; they didn't want to biopsy it for fear of pneumothorax (an abnormal collection of air or gas which may interfere with normal breathing). But my radiologist felt he'd have a pretty good chance of getting it.

I was certain it wasn't cancerous. I'd already gone four and a half years; I thought it had to be something else. But it did come back conclusive. I had stage IV cancer.

I felt that since they got the tumor out with the biopsy, there was no reason to get chemotherapy. In less than two months, the cancer grew into my paratracheal gland, so it was evident that I had to get chemo and get it fast. It was already four centimeters. So I scrambled and went to my local oncologist, a different one than I saw previously.

She said, "You better just make do with what you got and spend your time living the life that you have right now. It's growing so fast, and I don't think we'll be able to take care of it with chemotherapy."

I just sat there with my daughter and thought, *Are you kidding me? I just had lung surgery two months ago! I've still got fight in me. I guess I'll have to go to a research facility.*

My husband was having a hard time with my diagnosis, and we had split—the first of many troubles with our relationship. So my daughter and I went to Seattle Cancer Care, which is 122 miles away. We met a team of six physicians who told me they could give me some hope. We discussed it and decided hope is what we needed and we went for it!

It took about three hours to get to Seattle, and when I went, I was there all day. But it was worth it. Not only did I get the right treatment, they gave me hope. If your local oncologist doesn't give you hope, you might as well find your grave. It's that important.

From my experience, there's a big difference between quality of care at a research facility than the ones locally. Unlike when I got chemo locally, when I go to Seattle Cancer Care, they use sterile, surgical gloves. They also put you in a private room, so I'm not exposed to other people who have illnesses next to me.

I had a girlfriend who died from her port getting infected. And I saw a picture of her one day getting her port accessed with non-sterile gloves. The blue gloves are not sterile surgical gloves, the sterile ones are white. The port has direct access to your heart, and doctors are supposed to be using surgical gloves, but they're very expensive.

There were were little things I noticed. If I was going to fight this hard, I was going to make damn sure I got good care. So going the 122 miles is worth it for me, because I've never had a port infection.

They recommended a Phase 1 study using Abraxane, Avastin, and Taxol. After six months of twenty-four weekly treatments, I graduated to the second phase, where I received Tarceva. It was just horrible, so I voluntarily got off of that one. But then we had to find out what to do because it was still growing.

We decided that we were going to try a PARP inhibitor trial. I started with Cisplatin and Navelbene with the PARP inhibitor. By December 2011, I had a total response, so I continued on the PARP inhibitor only. I've had no evidence of disease ever since.

They're telling me that I will have to take this the rest of my life, every day. I'm accepting that's what I have to do in order to survive. For me it's more preventative than treatment, but it's still part of the Phase I clinical trial.

I've had a lot of side effects from my treatments. I can't really feel my left foot or leg because of neuropathy. I've experienced vomiting, extreme fatigue, and weight loss. I take a really good whole food vitamin, and I think that does wonders to alleviate side effects. I eat fresh fruit and vegetables, and I don't drink alcohol.

It's hard, to be honest. So I take it day by day, and that's helped me tremendously to get through. My triple-negative breast cancer support group has really been a godsend, and my friends and daughter are extremely supportive as well.

I take time to feel gratitude for what I have. God has blessed me with little things that help me get through. My dog Cody is an example. He'll get me out to take walks and knows when I'm having a hard time. Sometimes I'll fall asleep from exhaustion in the bathroom or on the sofa, and he wakes me up. It's amazing because he's just a little dog, but he's so smart.

I have a minister that comes and visits with me every week. My faith gives me strength and I believe is the reason I'm here. By all means, I really shouldn't be here. I feel it's a miracle, and there's a purpose to things.

Take the trial I'm on, for instance. There was a woman ahead of me who sadly passed away. And there have been people behind me who've have been pulled from the study because of relapses. All eyes are focused on me. They don't know what the drug is doing to me every day, but they do know it's keeping the cancer away.

Cancer has changed me. Before cancer, I would just listen to doctors, but now it's me making the decisions. I also take time to enjoy things that people take for granted—the sunset, rain, a dog licking my face, a baby smiling. If you don't know what pain is, sometimes you overlook the things that can bring you joy. And going through pain and agony has helped me slow down and look at those things. I needed to do that to help me smile and laugh.

I always try to make a positive out of a negative. I personally think that's a big factor in people who are doing well. They tend to be more positive and enjoy their lives instead of saying, "Why me? My life's a mess and I'm going to be depressed about it."

I think there are a lot of blessings in having cancer. I've met people who I never would have met before. I never would have realized how close I can become to God. I never believed in miracles before, but here I am, a living one.

Lessons Learned

- Listen to your spouse/significant other because they have fears, too. With everything going on, I probably didn't listen to my husband about his fears, even though I know he had them. Have discussions before it gets too involved.
- Consider clinical trials for targeted treatments, especially if you're triple negative. It can be grueling, but it can also offer you hope as opposed to regular chemo, which isn't targeted.
- It's important to manage side effects and not give up. With my trial, the first three treatments were hard to get through, but it gets easier as you go along. I encourage triple-negative stage IV patients (if all else has failed) to have their oncologist contact Abbott, the makers of the PARP inhibitor, to fight for compassionate use. At the very least, maybe that PARP will keep you from getting worse while they look for something else that will help you.

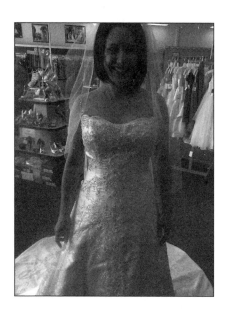

The Miracle Kid

BRITTANY ROSS
Boulder, CO
Age 27
Diagnosed in 2000 with Acute Myelogenous Leukemia (AML),
subtype M1

My story begins at the young age of fourteen. I started getting sick at the end of my eighth grade year in 1999 and it went into my freshman year of high school. I was coming down with all different kinds of illnesses that students get when they are in school together. I had horrible flus, colds, bronchitis, strep throat, allergies, and pink eye. My parents started taking me from one doctor to another, trying to get an answer to what could possibly be wrong with me.

I was at the children's hospital probably three to four times a week. I felt like a human pin cushion because I was getting poked and prodded constantly. Needles were and still are my number one phobia, so I was not the happiest teenage girl in the world. Unfortunately, everything that they tested and scanned me for returned as normal, and they said there was absolutely nothing to do. They prescribed antibiotics and sent me back home.

My sophomore year, I continued to get progressively sicker. About six weeks into the school year, I got shingles (an infection that causes a painful rash) all down the left side of my face. My brother-in-law Steven Eisenberg, an adult oncologist/hematologist who married my sister Julie just months previously, immediately knew what was wrong with me. He told my sister that kids just don't get shingles, and he was almost 100 percent sure I had leukemia.

He also knew, however, that my mom had lost her mother to metastatic breast cancer when she was in college and later lost her nine-year-old son Scott to a very rare complication from undiagnosed juvenile rheumatoid arthritis. So just in case he was wrong, he decided not to get us completely panicked right away. He told my sister he would watch me like a hawk, and if anything else happened, he would immediately take me in for testing.

On the morning of December 12, 2000, I woke up at 5:30 a.m. and immediately knew something was seriously wrong. My heart was racing, my head was pounding, my body was ice-cold, my vision was blurry, and I was so weak; I could not even stand up by myself. I was extremely pale and nauseated and felt like the room was spinning around in circles. I got down on my hands and knees and crawled into my parents' bedroom. My dad was out of town on a business trip at the time. I tried to pull myself onto the bed, but my voice was completely hoarse and I couldn't stop coughing and gagging.

In a loud whisper, I kept repeating, "Mommy, I'm going to be sick!" She quickly jumped out of bed and pushed me into the bathroom. My dizziness got a lot more intense, and I called out to her that I was about to faint. She got there in the nick of time, catching my head before it hit the tile floor. When I awoke, there were EMTs and paramedics surrounding me. I refused to let them take me to the hospital in the ambulance, so they carried me and laid me down in the backseat of my mom's car.

When we finally met with the doctor at the hospital, my mom told him everything that had been going on since the very beginning. He told my mom I was just dehydrated and ordered a blood draw and saline IV drip. About three hours after the nurse drew my blood, I noticed nobody bothered to send it to the lab to get it tested. The doctor signed my discharge papers and told my mom I should just go home, rest, have something to eat, drink plenty of fluids, and I would be fine.

Thank goodness I have such an extraordinary mom! She followed her mother's instinct and told him she absolutely would not take me home until she knew what was wrong with me. She told them to get my blood to the lab immediately. Reluctantly the doctor finally sent my blood to the lab. The results changed my whole world forever.

The blood labs showed 67 percent of the cells in my bone marrow had already become leukemic. My sister and her husband Steve, who was doing his fellowship at Georgetown University Hospital in Washington, DC, (where we lived at the time) came to the hospital right away. The hospital didn't have a pediatric oncology/hematology unit, so Steve told them to discharge me immediately so we could go to Georgetown, where he had arranged a room and meeting with the doctors in their pediatric unit.

My mom called my dad and my brother, who were living in Colorado. They both jumped onto the very first flight back to be at my side.

At Georgetown, doctors told my family I had Acute Myelogenous Leukemia (AML), an extremely aggressive form that is usually found in older adults. It only affects 500 to 1,000 kids worldwide per year. They told my parents that of all the kids and young adults diagnosed with AML, only 30 percent would make it to five years of remission and that the 70 percent would have recurrences or die within that time period. They gave me a 5 to 15 percent chance of survival and three weeks to live. I was about a month away from turning sixteen.

I didn't find out about my diagnosis until two days into treatment when my dad walked into my hospital room crying. His face was ashen white, and I asked him what was wrong. He sat down next to me in my bed, took my hand in his, and with tears in his eyes told me I had leukemia.

I already knew what leukemia was after watching movies like the *The Rainmaker*, and it hit me pretty hard. I knew my mom had already lost her mother and son to cancer. I was the final straw. I think she had my dad tell me because she wasn't ready to admit the truth or face up to it yet. Because I am the youngest in my family, I have always been Daddy's little princess. It broke my parents' hearts to watch me go through that.

When I first learned about my prognosis, my thoughts spiraled out of control. I worried I wouldn't see my family or friends again or get to graduate from high school or college. I told myself I wouldn't be able to get married and have my dream wedding or have a family of my own. I didn't even think I would live long enough to celebrate my sweet sixteen birthday, which was only a month away.

Once I came to terms with my diagnosis, I realized I needed to have a positive attitude. With my extraordinary support system, plus determination, persistence, stubbornness, and strong will to live, I knew I could beat this and survive. Quitting and giving up was not an option!

Steven oversaw all of my care and treatment and made sure the best decisions were being made on my behalf. That took a lot of the extra stressors off of me and my parents. I did two incredibly aggressive rounds of in-patient chemotherapy over a four-month period. Doctors told my parents they didn't expect me to ever be able to walk out of the hospital alive.

After being released from the hospital after each treatment, they told us that my bone marrow should begin to grow back in about thirty days. I was undergoing bone marrow aspirations and biopsies numerous times a week to see if anything had begun to grow back, but nothing. I was kept alive by being transfused with blood, antibiotics, and anything else they gave me. I would get to the outpatient clinic first thing in the morning and would be the very last one to leave at night. We did this for 275 days, to be exact. I also had two home nurses who came to our house several times a week to do blood draws.

My family was by my side every step of the way and there to help pull me through whatever was thrown our way. They slept on an air mattress by my hospital bed, and one of them was always there at all times. As I started to feel better, close family friends came to stay with me on the weekends so my parents were able to have time together and recover.

I think it was really hard for them to watch me go through so much sickness and pain. I know most of the time they felt pretty powerless. All they wanted to do was to make me better and they knew that it was out of their hands. But I knew they would do anything within their power to get me better and to make me stronger again. We worked as a team and created a bond that is truly unbreakable, and we came back stronger than ever.

My peers definitely treated me differently. When I was finally able to return to school, the school newspaper did a huge front page article about me. When I walked down the hallway—gaunt, bald, pale, and jaundiced—people stared, laughed, and pointed at me. They made fun of me and singled me out. People even said nasty things right to my face.

I quickly learned some really tough lessons at a very young age. I was no longer considered normal; I was the odd one who didn't fit in. People who I thought would be there for me disappeared completely. I knew the only people who I could really count on were my family, true friends, and my extraordinary medical team. It was tough, but I knew as long as I had my positive attitude and people who did support me, I would be okay and would survive.

My return to school would have been much more difficult without Marilyn Cox, my home-school tutor. She became my lifeline, guardian angel, and friend. She was incredible; together we managed to get me caught up even though we moved across the country and I was in three different high schools while battling cancer. I would never have been able to graduate without her and she continued to coach me and support me throughout college. She remains a very special person in my life today.

I was also extremely lucky to have friends in high places who created once-in-a-lifetime experiences for me to help keep my spirits up. One of our neighbors, Jared, was the director of entertainment at the MCI Center (now called Verizon Center) in Washington, DC. He got me front-row seats and sound check passes to every concert I wanted. I got to see and meet 'N Sync, 98 Degrees, and Rising. He even helped arrange for me to sit in the skybox when Michael Flatley came to town. I have been a dancer all my life, and Michael Flatley has always been one of my favorite dancers.

And our very dear family friend Andrea King, a Hollywood screen-writer, asked every movie studio for anything they weren't using to send to me in the hospital. The next thing I knew, I started getting packages from DreamWorks, Paramount, and other studios with things like autographed photos of actors and even copies of Academy Award–nominated movies that were still in theaters.

My room became known as "The Hollywood Room," and everybody—doctors, nurses, and patients—came into my room at mail time to see what I received. It gave me something to keep me going every single day and inspired me to never give up.

When I eventually recovered enough to travel, Andrea invited me and my family to come to California and took us to the set of *Sex and the City* (for which she had written episodes). We got to meet the actresses and sit next to Michael Patrick King to watch them film.

On my sixteenth birthday, she got some of my favorite stars to call me. Henry Winkler was the first. After our conversation, he started calling to check in on me every few weeks. When he was in Washington, DC, he took our family to lunch. They were probably some of the best hours of my life! He is one of the most kind, genuine, compassionate, and encouraging men I've ever known.

I believe having my medical team and this incredible support and encouragement made all the difference. Against all odds, I was declared in full remission on January 17, 2001, just four days after my sweet sixteen birthday. It was the best possible birthday present I ever could've imagined. I have been cancer-free ever since.

My doctors tell me I am truly one of kind—the only long-term AML survivor to still be alive and cancer-free (after only one month of chemotherapy) without undergoing any type of transplant. I am one in 6.5 billion, which is why I've earned the name, The Miracle Kid.

I have a new normal in my life now. My life will never ever return to the way that it was before getting my cancer diagnosis. I go in for a full blood workup about every six months, an annual bone density scan, and an EKG and an echocardiogram every two years. If I get sick or if something doesn't seem right, I'm always able to see my doctors. Like many childhood cancer survivors, I have many long-term side effects I will probably need to manage for the rest of my life. My immune system has been weakened, so I'm more susceptible to infections and have more trouble fighting them. I also deal with hypoglycemia, severe acid reflux, and circulation issues.

Emotionally I am pretty good most of the time, but I definitely have my bad moments. I have Asperger's Syndrome—a mild form of autism, but I am extremely high functioning. Sometimes I have severe anxiety and it can be an emotional roller coaster ride. Every single time I go to the doctor, I always have fear and anxiety because I worry easily.

There are constant reminders of my reality, but they help me to continue to be the woman I have become today. It's great to support other young people and their families who are going through the very same thing I experienced. I have been a motivational speaker and I have also done a ton of volunteer work with CureSearch for Children's Cancer,

Make-A-Wish Foundation, Stand Up 2 Cancer, Leukemia & Lymphoma Society, American Red Cross, American Cancer Society, Miracle Party Foundation and Physically Handicapped Actors and Musical Artists League (PHAMALY).

I give so much of my time because I realize I have been given a second chance at life. This is my opportunity to make a difference and to be a voice for others who can't do it for themselves. If I can make a difference in one person's life then I know that everything I've been through is well worth it.

Every young cancer survivor who has been a part of my life or who I have come into contact with has left a lasting impression on me. I love them like they are part of my family, and we share a bond that can't ever be broken. They are truly extraordinary human beings and a true gift to the world. They deserve to live full, healthy, and long lives like I have.

I know that to survive an illness you can't focus on statistics and what you're told. My success motto is, "The fight is 90 percent mental and 10 percent physical." I believe your attitude can dramatically affect the outcome and result. I've been told repeatedly the only reasons I continue to remain alive today are my positive attitude and support system. I chose to focus on things that made me happy and not dwell on bad things. My family reminded me all the time I was not a number, and I told them I refused to become another statistic. I wanted to defy the odds and prove the numbers wrong. I knew I had my whole entire life in front of me, and I would survive no matter what!

On September 28, 2013, I accomplished what my doctors said would be the "impossible dream" when my mom and dad walked me down the aisle to marry the love of my life. Patrick is my real-life Prince Charming. I am truly the luckiest woman in the world and am so happy to spend the rest of my life with him. We had an outdoor wedding at sunset so you could see the sun go down behind the mountains. It was absolutely magical, and the most special day of our lives.

My pediatric oncologist even flew in from Washington, DC, to Colorado to see me walk down the aisle. During the cocktail hour, my brother brought her over to take pictures with me. When I saw her walking toward me, I completely lost it and started bawling. Everything she had done for me and all of the moments of the last thirteen years came flooding back to me. I couldn't hold back the tears.

I truly can say cancer is the best thing that has happened to me. If I could go back and do it all over again, I would not change a single thing. I learned a lot of really tough lessons at a very young age that would've taken me a lot longer to learn had I not gone through cancer. I'm so glad I learned them because they helped shape the person I am today.

I try to see the good in every situation and not let little things get to me as much as they used to. I'm able to handle situations more responsibly and from a totally different perspective than I could have before. I cherish every single second I'm given and know every breath is a gift I no longer take for granted. I realize now that pretty much everything in life is a privilege, not a right.

This experience has taught me I am capable of more than I thought I was. If I could fight cancer and face death at the age of fifteen, there's really nothing I can't handle. There's no longer a reason for me to be afraid of death, though I'm not ready to go yet.

My family and I have a wonderful guru we follow, Sai Maa, who talks about having a purpose and giving love even in the worst possible circumstances. I guess my purpose has not been fulfilled yet because I'm still here. I knew thirteen years ago it was not my time to go.

Lessons Learned

- Cherish every single moment you have been given to be with the people you love and who love you.
- In the time you have been given, live your life to the absolute fullest and accomplish everything you have ever hoped to do.
- Be grateful and make sure you tell the people in your life how much you love them. Let them know how important and special they are to you each and every day.

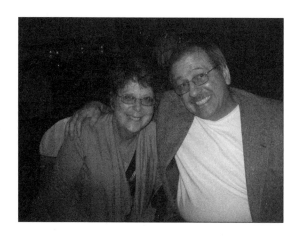

Still Making It Work . . . Sixteen Years Later

CAROLE KUBRIN
Cincinnati, OH
Age 57
Living with stage IV, HER2-positive breast cancer since 1998

When I was working as a special education teacher, I always felt my students were my kids. My resource room became a place where they could come and let off steam. They could tell me their frustrations and we could work together to solve or strategize how we'd make it work. And that's what I told myself when I felt a lump in 1995 and learned that I had stage I breast cancer: "We're going to make this work."

I had a lumpectomy and was sent home. My husband, Ed, told people I had breast cancer, and I said, "No I don't, because they took the tumor out, so it's all gone." That's how naive I was. I taught at a Catholic school and they had Wednesday mass in the mornings, so I scheduled my chemo around that. I would finish up right before lunch and then I'd go back to school and finish out the day. After that was done, I had radiation therapy. They gave me a clean bill of health and put me on the hormone therapy drug Tamoxifen as a preventative measure.

Three years later, while I was teaching and finishing up my Masters program at Xavier University, I had this jarring pain in my left rib underneath where I had the lumpectomy, so I finally had a chest X-ray done. It was during the holidays, and I was going to take my daughters—Lauren, who was in fifth grade, and Tricia, in third grade—and their friends to the mall. But I scheduled an appointment with my primary doctor to discuss my test results, so we stopped there first. I went in and he told me I had metastases on the bone.

He said that I could take my time processing the news. When he came back in, he said, "You're holding yourself together pretty well." I responded "Well, I've got this group of girls out here who I've got to take somewhere, so I have to hold it together." The cancer was back, but it wasn't going to interfere with our lives—not yet. And we went to the mall.

We were all a mess and it wasn't a "happy New Year" for us.

Several days later, I had a CT scan and went to see my oncologist, Dr. Bechhold, for my results. I walked in and said, "Yeah, I know the cancer's back in my bone." And she told me, "So, you know about the liver?" There was the punch in the stomach I didn't see coming.

Years later, Ed told me the nurse had taken him aside and told him he needed to get my affairs in order. He didn't tell me about it at the time, and luckily they didn't share that with me. They just said to me, "We're going to fight this." And that's all I heard. No one ever gave me stats on how long they thought I had. Even if they did, I would have proven them wrong!

I was shocked, but was able to discuss our game plan. She suggested a stem cell transplant. They were still doing them for breast cancer patients at that time.

The next week I had my port put in, and that afternoon I started high-dose chemo to get ready for the stem cell transplant. Right away, my mindset was that we were going to fight this. I kept working because I needed that normalcy. I didn't have a full-time class; I was more of a tutor. I probably wouldn't have been able to work if I'd had a self-contained class.

But I hit a glitch when a study came out saying the results for stem cell for breast cancer patients were the same as with high-dose chemo. Insurance companies refused to pay for stem cell transplants anymore. I went through the three levels of appeals, and one of their doctors looked at my case and said they would only pay for chemo. I went all the way to their appeals board and had to hire a lawyer and take out a second mortgage to fight it. Throughout my battle, I continued to do the chemo.

It just wasn't right to have people look at your records without knowing you are refusing treatment because they're looking at their bottom line. I swore I would fight this all the way up to the top. I even had my congressman call the company. I don't know what did it, but they finally changed their minds and agreed to pay for the stem cell transplant.

I had it done in September—four months later than we planned. I took time off from school through December. I did alright with it, but there were times I felt pretty low and started thinking, "Am I going to survive this?" I didn't want my girls to see me like that, so I limited my pity parties.

After the procedure, I went back to teaching and started on the aromatase inhibitor Arimadex and then Aromasin. Scans showed spots on my lungs, but they would disappear, so the medicine seemed to be working.

In 2003, they found a small tumor by my bile duct, and they couldn't determine whether or not it was cancer. So I went in and had a lobectomy. They took out the right part of my liver plus my gallbladder and fixed all that up. That's when they found out that I was HER2-positive, and then they put me on Herceptin and Aredia for the bones.

The next year, I was so weak and tired and my muscle tone was so poor, I had a hard time walking. It was so bad that I applied for retirement disability. I didn't want to give in, but I didn't think I could do my job effectively anymore, so I was done teaching at the end of the school year. That summer I found out I had hyperthyroidism, which was causing my problems, so I had radiation, which put the thyroid in check.

After receiving my mammogram results, they wanted to move up my testing from one year to every six months. I felt I had to try something else. I started seeing a naturopathic doctor and taking supplements, doing acupuncture, and changing my diet. I was doing well and was scared of chemicals, so I stopped using Aredia and Herceptin. I thought they already did their job and all the naturopathic stuff would keep it at bay. I felt so good that in 2006, I reapplied to teach again and got my job back.

At the same time all of this was happening, Ed was diagnosed with multiple sclerosis (MS). I always thought, "I'm glad that I'm the one who had the cancer because I don't think I'd be able to take care of it if someone else had it." Sometimes I'm not the most patient caregiver. I want to say, "Just do it! I got through this, so you can get through this, too." It's hard being on the other end of it. But I know this is what we've been dealt, and we just have to be strong for each other.

In September 2008, I started slowing down again. I couldn't eat or walk as well, and one night I started throwing up blood. So I went into the emergency room, and that's when they told me the cancer was back in my liver. It wasn't looking good, and I was a mess. I argued back and forth with the oncologist on call, saying the cancer wasn't back, and he assured me it was. They had me on Vicodin, which made me loopy, and I didn't even know what was going on. Lauren later told me, "Don't you remember? You were so mean to people." I didn't remember anything.

The girls were pretty shaken up this time, too. At that point, life revolved around the cancer. People were bringing meals and doing things for us. We tried to create a sense of normalcy and told them, "We're going to get through this."

When all this happened, I decided to quit working with the naturopath. My family told me, "This stuff's going out, you're done. We're back on the chemical route." Now, all I take are multivitamins and a probiotic. I'm leery of anything else.

I went back on chemo, getting Taxotere and Herceptin. After one treatment, my blood counts got so low that I needed a plasma transfusion. Dr. Bechhold said to me, "You know, maybe it's time to start thinking about hospice." As she started talking to me, I just felt myself getting stronger and knowing that we weren't calling hospice, we were calling my church. My feet started tapping and I knew I had to get out of there because I had some calls to make! My doctor was very surprised to see me walking out of the building instead of being pushed in a wheelchair. That night, I had church members pray over me.

Since my white blood counts were so low, she suggested we stop the Taxotere until my counts improved and to continue with Herceptin. I responded so well to the Herceptin; my tumor markers went from over 1,000 down to near normal levels. I never did go back on Taxotere! That's when Dr. Bechhold said, "Don't even think about going off of Herceptin ever again." And I've been taking it, along with Xgeva for the bones, ever since.

Our family always has been about being strong. Eventually, I got better and we got to the point where we laughed about it. Our family motto is, "Humor can get you through a whole mess of ugly!" We didn't make cancer the front and center of our lives. We always tried to downplay it and not even think about it. Cancer is something we have to deal with, but we're not going to pity ourselves or worry about it all the time. We just kept plugging along. Our attitude is, "It might not be great right now, but let's wait an hour maybe, it'll improve and things will look better."

I feel we were surrounded by angels, and that helped. Friends were always willing to step up to do things for us. And there were so many people—some I didn't even know—who prayed for me.

I don't know if I was naive, but I always thought I was going to get better. When Dr. Bechhold walked in the room, I asked what we were going to do to fight it, and that's what we did together. I'm not always a follow-through person, but it just seemed like I had this strength and spirit that came out whenever I heard bad news. I would come out and be ready to do battle.

Life is about living, not worrying about when you're going to die. A doctor has never told me, "You've got three months," or "You've got six months." I never wanted to hear that because they don't know; they're just making a guess. The times I have good test results, I'll point to the ceiling and I'll say, "Dr. Bechhold, I know somebody up there," and she'll say, "Don't I know it. You are an inspiration because I see how hard you've fought all this."

Sometimes self-doubt creeps in and I wonder if I have asked for too many miracles. But I think I'm like everyone else. I wanted to see my girls graduate high school. Then I wanted to see them graduate college. Once that happened, I wanted to live to see them get married and have babies. I keep reaching for all those milestones. I was able to see my oldest daughter get married and now I'm waiting for those grandkids and having another wedding to plan! No pressure, girls!

I'm grateful I am here to see my daughters have successful careers. Tricia's working at a law firm in DC, using Japanese she learned while teaching in Japan. And Lauren is carrying on the work I did teaching special needs kids in my school. When I went to file my papers for my disability retirement, Lauren had just graduated from Ohio State with a degree in special education. She took my papers to my school and she said to them, "I'm a special education graduate; if you need a person, I can fill in." So they said, "Sure, you got the job." She's been teaching there ever since. And last year, Ed and I were able to go to Japan and visit with Tricia. That's something we can cross off our bucket list!

I still have spots in my bones, and they're keeping a close eye on me. I struggle sometimes with pain, but I'm still here. I do have my moments. Sometimes I wrap myself around prayer blankets and talk to God, asking for the reason I'm around when so many other people haven't survived. I'll say, "They were doing so much more for others and for breast cancer . . . why am I still here?"

I think the reason I'm here is to tell my story because that's what God wants me to do—to show people there are miracles in life. He's given me a boatload of them and my mission is to tell people that and to be an inspiration to newly diagnosed people with stage IV cancer. When women hear how many years I have survived with stage IV breast cancer, their look of surprise changes to one of determination. A look that says, "I can, too!"

People will look at our family and say, "You people have gone through so much." Yeah, we have, but we can show you can get through it.

Lessons Learned

- Don't let fear get in the way of learning about your disease and treatment. I didn't always research enough because I'd end up reading about poor survival rates; I couldn't deal with that. So I kept the information at a high level. I didn't do scans all the time in the beginning, and that worked against me because the cancer had metastasized. I wanted to dwell on the positive, but at the risk of knowing the truth.

- Statistics are just numbers. My story is individual and unique, and who knows how long I have to live? I do think it was a good thing I avoided looking at statistics about poor survival rates. Instead I focused on how to deal with what was going on in the moment and where to go from there.

- Share your experience and hope, rather than give advice. I don't tell people with cancer it will be okay, because I don't know that. I just tell them my story and say, "This is how I did it and how we tried to stay strong." That's the only hope that I can really give anybody.

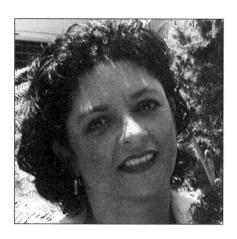

Breaking Down Barriers

DAKOTA NEAL
Sacramento, CA
Age 54
Diagnosed in 2009 with stage IV Leiomyosarcoma

We come from humble beginnings. I came from a family of seven children, and I'm the only girl. We went through a lot of hard times, but I was very determined and strong-willed. In school, I was always a strong student because I wanted to be successful.

My mom divorced my father when I was about eight, and she had six children at the time. It was tough for her being a single mom but we had to figure out how to make it work and pull together as a family unit. My mom remarried when I was thirteen, but until then I had to step in and take the role of caretaker for my younger brothers as my mom had to go to work.

I learned so much from my mother. I think she's an amazing person. Her children have always been so important to her, and she has had to overcome such adversity. My mother is caucasian and my father is African American. They met when my dad was stationed in England. My mother was very protective of us and told us we needed to be strong because there was a lot of non-acceptance of interracial marriages and biracial children.

Today, being biracial is accepted. Back in the '60s it wasn't, and I didn't feel fully embraced by either race, although I felt more accepted by the African American community. My mother taught us to block out all the negativity and move forward. She often said, "Life isn't always fair, and people don't always see the inside. Don't worry about other people. Just know who you are inside and be that person."

Her lessons served me well when I started experiencing symptoms leading to my cancer diagnosis. It was 2005, I was forty-six, married, and had two young children, Simone and Sterling, who were six and twelve years old. And I just changed jobs, working for the State of California. It was a very stressful time both at work and at home, and to add to the stress, my thirty-nine-year-old brother passed away unexpectedly.

I started noticing an aching, throbbing pain in my tibia. I passed it off, thinking I injured my ankle when I bumped it as I was rushing around one day. A couple of months later, it wouldn't go away and it started to wake me up at night. So I went to the doctor. They told me just to stay off my feet and rest.

The pain persisted, and I continued to go to my doctor for about a year until finally I told him, "Don't you think you need to do an X-ray?" He replied, "Oh, we never X-rayed it?" So they did an X-ray and saw a huge tumor that went from right below my knee to my ankle. It covered the whole tibia.

When they initially biopsied it, they determined it was just a giant cell-benign tumor. I had surgery to take out the bone and replace it with an internal prosthetic. When the surgeon looked at the inside of the tumor, he knew it had to be cancer. The pathology report confirmed it was some type of sarcoma.

My specimen underwent five different biopsies before they determined I had leiomyosarcoma, a very rare sarcoma. Usually it affects the uterus or other soft tissue, not the bone. One biopsy determined it was osteosarcoma (bone cancer). Three others indicated it was leiomyosarcoma. They did another biopsy, which indicated osteosarcoma. They finally said, "We've been messing around way too long. Let's treat you aggressively." They suggested amputating my leg.

My mom and husband Brian were upset over the prospect of my losing my leg, but I said, "I'm going to fight it as aggressively as I can because I have young children, and I need to be here. Let's amputate my leg. There are a lot of people with prosthetics. I'm fortunate; a lot of people are in a worse situation than this."

After I recovered from surgery, my surgeon referred me to an oncologist in Sacramento, but the oncologist basically told me there was nothing he could do. I went back to my surgeon who said, "That's not correct. You need to go see a sarcoma specialist."

He referred me to a specialist, Dr. Sant Chawla in Santa Monica, which is about four hundred miles away from where I live. When we went there, he said, "If you had been diagnosed with this three or four years ago, you'd have had a life expectancy on average of about six months, but there are so many new drugs now. You need to be on a treatment plan right away."

I went to a doctor at Stanford, which is closer, for a second opinion. She told us Dr. Chawla was a wonderful sarcoma specialist, so we got right back in the car and went down to Santa Monica to start treatment. Dr. Chawla said, "We're going to treat you as aggressively as we can. You're young and healthy." The regimen I underwent consisted of, over a period of time, Ifex (Ifosfamide), Taxotere, Gemzar, Adriamycin, and Cisplatin, and then interferon and Zometa. It was hard for our family, because it's a seven-hour drive from Sacramento to Santa Monica. My husband drove and my mom watched the kids.

We stayed in a hotel since I had to wear a chemo bag for five days, twenty-four hours a day. I would take two weeks off of work and then

I'd go back for another five or six days. We both tried to work while we were there; it helped to keep our minds busy.

Before being diagnosed with cancer, I never took one sick day in my entire twenty-year career. I never even had a cold! My boss joked, "Couldn't you have started with a cold, Dakota? How do you go from never being sick to having cancer?"

It was difficult, but I stayed positive and knew I was going to fight this with everything I had. I didn't think my diagnosis was a death sentence. I didn't want my kids to get stressed. I thought if I stayed positive, my kids would see that and wouldn't be stressed about it. I always told my kids we had a fighting chance, and that I'd be fighting with every breath to be there for them. My daughter had a hard time with me losing my leg. She didn't want other kids looking at me and would get mad at them if they did, but overall, I think she handled it well.

When I went into the infusion room, I'd say to patients, "We're going to fight this!" And they'd say, "Oh, I think that cancer's afraid of you Dakota!" That was my mindset. I didn't look at any statistics; I never even looked my cancer up online, because I felt I wasn't a statistic. I would follow my doctor's orders, eat healthy, and have faith. I only watched happy shows on TV. I even stopped watching medical programs on television because it was stressing me out. I made myself eat when I had no appetite, drink water when the thought of drinking more water made me nauseated, and got dressed and out of bed every day. By the end of 2007, life seemed to be getting back to normal.

In November 2009, I started having pain in my back and my spine. I had an X-ray, CT scan, and MRI, which didn't show anything. I kept saying, "No, I feel something. I know that pain." I had a physician, Dr. Kenneth Wiesner, who was my advocate, and he kept sending me for studies until we finally discovered a tumor hidden in the spine. They did a biopsy and diagnosed it as a recurrence of leiomyosarcoma.

I thought I had this beat, but obviously I didn't, so I thought, *Okay, we did this once; we're going to do this again. One step at a time, let's go for it.* Rather than looking in the mirror and wondering why this was happening to me, I thought about how I was going to live my life going forward and how my kids were going to see me. If something were to happen to me, how did I want them to remember me? I thought, *What if I only have a short time to live and my kids remember me as being depressed and negative and not having faith and the fight?* I wanted to show them how to deal with obstacles that may come their way later in life.

So I surrounded myself with positive people and things that made me happy. When I started getting into a funk, I figured out something to do like going shopping with my daughter, having my husband take me for a ride, watching my favorite movie, or talking to a friend. Sometimes I chose to go into prayer and meditation. I didn't want to go to what I call "the dark side."

Dr. Chawla gave me chemo and then sent me to Stanford for radiation, where I was again fortunate to have great doctors, Dr. Sara Donaldson and Dr. Steven Chang. I underwent chemo with Dr. Chawla and went back to Stanford for cyberknife radiation, which uses a robot to guide radiation straight to the tumor. After that procedure, I had twenty-one days of traditional radiation on my back, and then went back to Santa Monica for more chemo.

I was diligent about my follow-up care, and I was fine until a CT scan showed that it had recurred in my lungs in June of 2010. Dr. Chawla was heading a trial and he put me in it. The trial drug was called Yondelis. Every six weeks I had a CT scan, and the tumor shrank each time. In December, Stanford removed the portion of my lung where the tumor was located and found all the cancers cells were dead. My oncologist said the chemo/Yondelis killed the cancer.

I received a few more treatments of Yondelis and went back on interferon and Zometa for maintenance until July 2013. I've had no evidence of disease since.

I was very blessed through this journey because I had a strong support system. My husband drove me to every single procedure and treatment.

He read with me and cooked healthy meals every night. I also had my mom, who would do anything and everything possible to help. And I had lots of friends who would come and take me for coffee or lunch or encourage me to exercise. My best friend from childhood was diagnosed with breast cancer within a few days of my being diagnosed, so we went through chemo together.

And my kids, they kept me going, too. When I came home tired from chemo, my son would play piano for hours and hours until I fell asleep. What a blessing!

Because I've received so much support, I try to give back to others when I can. I started going to an AME church that a friend recommended and met Reverend Tammie Denyse, who is a breast cancer survivor. She founded an organization called Carrie's Touch Inc., which provides education, outreach, support, and advocacy for breast cancer survivors with emphasis on the African American community. I really believed in the organization and its purpose, so I decided to volunteer as their treasurer.

Cancer is cancer. It's a fight that touches a lot of people, whether it's breast cancer, a sarcoma, or prostate cancer. We all have families, dreams, and ups and downs in our lives, so we have to give back. When another person is down, you need to pick them up, and I believe you are blessed in return.

I think the African American community is a little more reserved about cancer. Many people don't want to talk about it; it's taboo. I think people are more likely to talk to me about my cancer because it's a physical condition they can see. A lot of people initially think I lost my leg through an accident or diabetes, so they will feel more comfortable asking me what happened, and a conversation about cancer follows. My oncologist sometimes asks me to talk to people at the clinic who have been diagnosed with a sarcoma. A mom of a little girl who had bone cancer wanted me to talk to her about it. She was so strong, she inspired me. And I've had a lot of people ask me to just sit and talk to somebody that had been recently diagnosed with cancer.

I share my experience so they know that there is hope. I'll say, "Cancer took my leg, but life is good. I'm blessed and I'm going forward and living my life. Cancer can take my limb, but it can't take who I am as a person. It's not gonna hold me down!"

Having cancer has changed my life in many ways. I was always a believer, but I think going through this process strengthened my faith. Before I had cancer, I considered myself Christian, but I didn't think too much about it. Besides my children, I don't think I ever prayed for anything. But throughout my diagnosis and treatment, I found myself praying for strength, health, and to be there for my children. I told myself it was going to be alright no matter how it turned out. I knew a lot of this was out of my control, but I was going to do my part and knew God would work through my doctors to heal me and help me cope.

I have different priorities in life now. I see myself more as someone living in a community as opposed to just my family unit. Cancer has made me realize we're all one and in this journey together. I'm more outspoken about negative behavior and people judging other people's lives because you never know what another person is going through.

It's also changed the way I relate to my kids. My son is very artistic, but before I was diagnosed, I was focused on his grades so he could be successful in life. I was trying to fit my kids into a mold I thought they should be in. Now I say, "As long as you are happy with who you are as a person—you are a good person and doing your best to be a productive part of society—you're successful." It's not about being materialistic or "keeping up with the Joneses." You have one life; follow your dreams.

My life is very busy. My daughter is in high school now and plays water polo and sings in the choir. We enjoy going to her tournaments and music programs. I spend a lot of time studying my family's geneal-ogy. It fascinates me, and I think it helps me unwind after work. I've looked into both my European and African ancestry.

I feel like I'm a lot more centered and happy in many ways than I was before I had cancer. Since tomorrow's not promised to any of us, I continue to do what is mine to do and let go of things I can't control. None of us know what our journey holds. It's not necessarily what happens to us, it's how we handle what happens to us that matters.

Lessons Learned

- Fight with everything you have and don't look at statistics or what has happened to others. We're all individuals, not statistics.
- Listen to your body and know when you're tired or feel something is wrong. It can be telling you to get more rest or to check with a doctor.
- Surround yourself with a good team of doctors and don't be afraid to get a second opinion. Make sure you continue to follow up with your care.
- And most of all, remember happiness is a choice. Try to find something that makes you smile and gives you purpose and have faith that things will get better.

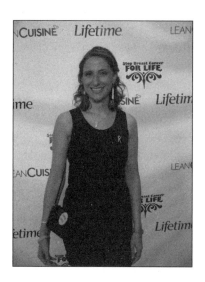

Helping and Healing

DIKLA BENZEEVI
Los Angeles, CA
Age 44
Living with stage IV, HER2-positive breast cancer since 2002

I was born in Israel. My dad was an economic advisor for the World Bank with projects all over the world. Our family moved every few years. We lived in Greece, the Philippines, and the tiny island of Saipan, near Guam. I loved Saipan the most because it was a tropical paradise and my best friends were my next-door neighbors. It was so small and beautiful. Everything was an adventure. My best friends and I would play together all the time—baseball, jump rope, and braiding each other's hair. Typhoons and hurricanes came through, yet I was never scared. We'd board up the windows and get to stay home from school. We'd swim at the beautiful white sand beaches and enjoy the warm weather year round.

We moved to Irvine, California, when I was ten. It was weird for me to stay in one place. After two years, I thought, *Where are we moving to next?* Little did I know there would be so many storms to brave right here in California.

My mother was diagnosed with breast cancer when I was twelve, and passed away when I was fourteen. A year later, my dad was diagnosed with colon cancer. This happened in the early to mid '80s when there weren't all the cancer support services there are now. We did not share the news about my mom's ordeal with anyone outside the family. It was a very difficult time coping with the trauma of my mom's illness and suffering and the uncertainty it created for our future as a family unit. Since we were new to the country, my mom's medical care was out-of-pocket. Two years of treatments and surgeries bankrupted us. All the savings my parents had built up over the decades went down the drain. Our home fell apart when my mom passed away; she was our foundation.

My dad moved back to Israel to receive his cancer treatment because that is where he had his pension, Social Security, and health insurance. I moved in with two of my three older brothers. They went from being young adults, figuring out college and what they were going to do with their lives, to being caretakers and making very adult decisions. It was a crazy time.

I think we just survived day-to-day. It took many years to learn how to live with some kind of peace of mind. We had to go to school and figure out how to pay bills. We worried about our dad, and I'm sure he was worried about us. He would come and visit every year.

I went to college when I was sixteen to study biology. Because of our family's experience, I wanted to work in cancer research. I was able to pay for college through loans, grants, and working two to four jobs at a time. I picked up coping mechanisms that probably weren't the healthiest, and suppressed my feelings because I didn't have time to deal with them. It felt like if I let them come out, I would become depressed and unable to function.

After I graduated from college, I went to Israel to learn more about my culture and to spend time with my dad. I really didn't know my dad was so ill. I moved in with him and realized he was going through chemo and radiation for terminal colon cancer. He and my brothers had not told me, trying to protect me from worry and concern. Going to chemo with him seemed so surreal to me. Dad was in a lot of pain the last four years of his life. His cancer had spread and pinched a nerve in his leg, and he had this awful sciatica pain that no painkillers could really manage. He paced the apartment for hours, shuffling with his cane, because sitting still would hurt him more. It broke my heart. We had a lot of family there and he had a good social circle, but to watch my dad endure so much pain and suffering was awful.

As a caregiver, the torture in my soul was horrendous—first my mom, then my dad. What I desperately wanted for them was something no one could offer: to eliminate their cancer, pain and suffering, and return them to the vital, vibrant, and healthy parents they deserved to be. I wish I had been diagnosed first because then I would have had a better understanding of what a person going through cancer needed and wanted. I did my best, but I felt I wasn't taking all the right steps to providing the support and care my parents needed.

I worked long hours in a cancer research lab until my dad entered hospice care. I couldn't deal with lab work anymore after his death because I didn't want to deal with anything related to cancer. So I worked as a legal secretary, and took it easy in comparison to my previous schedule. I worked regular hours and expanded my social life.

I stayed in Israel for three years and then came back to Los Angeles, where I worked at a talent agency for several years. I saw a lot of celebrities—Jennifer Lopez, John Travolta, Liam Neeson, and others. It was very exciting, busy work.

I was working at Paramount Pictures when I was diagnosed. I had no symptoms. With my family history, I knew that when I turned forty, I'd need to be very conscientious about getting mammograms and performing breast self-exams. But I was thirty-two; I didn't consider breast cancer in my world at all.

It was August 2002 when I went for my annual exam and my gynecologist felt something in my breast. She said it was probably a cyst, but sent me to a breast center to get it examined. I didn't think much of it. In hindsight, I was fortunate. A lot of my young cancer survivor friends had doctors who had brushed off their concerns without further examination, or ended up being later diagnosed with tumors that had gotten larger, and/or with cancer that had spread.

I went to a breast center in Van Nuys where I had my first mammogram, ultrasound, and four stereotactic biopsies on both of my breasts. I was so clueless. I thought, *Why in the hell are we going through this? I'm missing all this work. Can we just get this done so I can get back to work?* Later, the radiologist called me from the breast center and asked me to come in to discuss the results. I was worried about another day off from work. My brother and his wife offered to come to the appointment with me. I wondered why they were going to drive three hours to go with me. I guess I thought company would be nice. I was so naive.

At the appointment, the radiologist told us I had cancer in my right breast. It was like all the sound got sucked from the room. I didn't know how to take this information. I heard it, but it wouldn't absorb. I felt and looked fine. I had no breast cancer symptoms. Nothing had changed in my life to warrant the diagnosis. I couldn't even feel the lump in my breast.

I don't remember being afraid of dying. I just didn't know what to think or expect. I didn't think, *Am I going to die like my parents?* I was scared about my job security, how much work I was going to miss, and how I would take care of myself. I didn't want to suffer like my parents did. When they had chemo, they didn't have access to the anti-nausea drugs we have today.

I took time off from work because I had so many doctor appointments. I saw oncologists, social workers, and surgeons who were telling me different things and all their words didn't make sense to me.

I had a biology background, though granted this had been many years earlier. For me, the terminology surrounding a breast cancer diagnosis and treatment was like learning a new language. I felt enormous pressure to become an instant expert in all things breast cancer in a very short amount of time. I researched and read for weeks with a certain, if not desperate, vigor to understand it all. I felt very overwhelmed. There were days I didn't want to do anything; the burden was too much.

My brothers were very supportive. One brother who lived near me helped a lot. Another brother is an ER doctor, and he helped me stay levelheaded and guided me on to the next steps. His wife and kids were of great support and comfort. My third brother was overseas for work, and he moved back immediately. My siblings knew and had lived through what my parents went through and wanted to minimize it happening to me. It was a very scary time.

Because I had such a strong family history of breast cancer, I was tested to see if I had the BRCA hereditary gene mutations. The BRCA tests came back negative.

During the six weeks after my diagnosis, I went to three or four hospitals to get opinions. They did CT, PET MRI, and bone scans. The biopsies showed I had estrogen receptor (ER), progesterone receptor (PR), and HER2-positive breast cancer. In addition to the large breast tumor, the scans showed a small spot in a vertebra in my spine. They called it a bone cyst. No one considered it anything to worry about, so I was diagnosed with stage III rather than stage IV metastatic breast cancer. Only one hospital guaranteed to give me the targeted cancer treatment drug Herceptin, a drug specific for HER2-positive breast cancer. The others offered clinical trials where I might or might not get Herceptin. I chose to go to the first hospital. In addition, I was about to start carboplatin and Taxotere chemotherapy. I chose to start Herceptin and chemo before having breast surgery to shrink the tumors and hopefully have a less extensive breast surgery later. After four of six rounds of chemo and after scans revealed a dramatic shrinkage in my breast tumor size, I had a lumpectomy and lymph node dissection performed, after which I finished my remaining rounds of chemo and Herceptin.

About a week before I started chemo, I found out treatment could affect my fertility. I was very upset that no one had mentioned this or at least told me what to do to try to protect my fertility. I wasn't in a relationship at the time, but I wanted the option to have children in the future.

Within a week I learned about egg freezing and rushed around trying to find a clinic to get information. I realized, after my consult at one clinic, that it wasn't too late to do egg freezing since I hadn't started treatment. They told me they would have to give me a lot of estrogen to induce multiple egg releases during my next cycle. I would have to delay starting my cancer treatment until the next menstrual cycle happened. I feared that waiting another four weeks and getting pumped full of estrogen would most likely make my cancer grow and spread and get worse. At the time, the success rate with egg freezing was only 17 percent and this was in a lab in Italy. Because of the high health risks and low probability outcome for success, I decided against undergoing the egg freezing procedure. This was a difficult decision for me as I weighed all my treatment options for long-term survivorship and fertility preservation.

Over the last several years, successful egg-freezing techniques have improved dramatically. There is a lot more information available for women now regarding the various fertility preservation methods they can try through groups like Fertile Hope and Fertile Action. These groups were not around when I was diagnosed. More doctors are now discussing the effects of treatments on fertility and fertility preservation options with young women right at the time of diagnosis. At the time I was diagnosed, few doctors were cognizant of the need to discuss these topics. From the few choices I had available to try to preserve my fertility during chemotherapy, I chose ovarian suppression therapy.

After nearly a year of treatment, including surgery and radiation, I started on Tamoxifen. In the summer of 2004, I started experiencing back pain. By the fall, the pain became unbearable, so I had a bone scan. It showed the spine lesion they previously thought was a bone cyst was indeed a tumor. It had flared up since 2002 and had grown very quickly since I finished my initial treatments in 2003, so much so that it fractured my vertebra. They had misdiagnosed me at first; I was actually stage IV the whole time. If they had diagnosed this spine tumor correctly, they could have kept me in active treatment continuously so the spine tumor would not have grown and fractured my vertebra, and likely would have been controlled.

I lost a year of my life because of the spine tumor. The tumor threatened my spinal cord. The cancer grew so fast, there was barely anything keeping the vertebra together. My doctors were concerned I would end up paralyzed. A few days after I received my scan results, they put me in a chin-to-waist back brace to stabilize my spine. I became fully disabled and wasn't allowed to move much. Dealing with the spine tumor led to a very long recovery process.

When I was previously going through chemo, I tried to maintain some semblance of independence. I felt like crap, but I drove and went to work. Now in a back brace I needed help with everything. It was a fifteen-minute process to get in the shower. I wasn't able to bend over or lift anything over five pounds, so I couldn't do laundry or get things from the fridge. The only time I could take the brace off was when I laid down.

My brothers and their families helped me tremendously, but I knew I couldn't place all the responsibility on them. By that time, I had gone to support groups, so I reached out to everyone I knew, both in the cancer community and outside it—about one hundred people. Ten people stepped up big time and volunteered to help with groceries, laundry, and rides to appointments. They were busy professionals, but they would tell me when they were available.

The chin-to-waist back brace made my cancer very evident. Everyone asked what happened. I thought, *Do I go through a thirty-minute explanation or do I make up a story of a hang gliding or mountain climbing accident?* That would be more exciting and fun than telling them the truth.

I use dark, dry humor to cope a lot. A good friend of mine, Bonnie, who has since passed away, helped me tremendously with a lot of things I had to do. When we went shopping together for clothes, we'd use the handicap dressing room and she'd have to pull down my pants to help me change. You should have seen it! I had to lean against the wall like I was being arrested and getting a pat-down. I don't even know what people outside were thinking. It made me laugh when people said I seemed inches taller because the back brace made me stand straighter and have better posture. Bonnie even kindly embroidered for me on a long sleeve jean shirt the words "I'm too sexy for my brace." Humor and compassionate support from others helped me persevere and cope with a long-term difficult situation.

I hated feeling so helpless, but it was a huge learning experience. It forced me to reveal my vulnerability to people and not be stubborn about asking for help. I didn't have a choice. People were very kind-hearted. In my mind, I didn't want to be a burden to anyone and only wanted to help others. I had to swallow a huge piece of humble pie and accept help.

I made a lot of great friends from this time. People revealed their caring, compassionate nature. A lot of people who I didn't know well stepped up; they were acquaintances. To me, accepting help was very uncomfortable, but I realized that these were wonderful individuals who volunteered and wanted to help. Receiving and accepting help from people I knew and from virtually "strangers" was a huge, positive learning experience.

Finally, in the spring of 2005, I had a vertebrectomy (spine fusion surgery) to remove the tumor. It was major surgery. The surgeons deflated my left lung, and went through the side of my body and in through the front of the spinal column to scoop out the tumor. Then they put in a carbon fiber cage, took out a piece of my rib, ground it up, and filled the carbon fiber cage with my rib powder. This is held in place with titanium screws and rods.

Before the surgery, they told me they didn't know how it would turn out. I could end up paralyzed, have chronic numbness, or be in chronic pain the rest of my life. I put together advanced directives because I knew I could die from the effects of the surgery or the cancer. Luckily the tumor was in the thoracic vertebrae, which does not bend much in normal, everyday movement. I wouldn't and didn't feel the loss in mobility as I would have if the surgery was in my cervical and lumbar spine where one bends more. The surgery was a success. I spent the rest of 2005 recovering.

I was in remission for a while which felt great and was a huge relief, then scans in 2006 showed spots in my lungs. My doctor considered them to be scar tissue from my spine surgery, but they started growing larger. Finally in 2007, the spots were diagnosed as lung metastases. My breast cancer had spread to my lungs. I was scared and overwhelmed. What did this diagnosis mean to my longevity, my quality of life, and my chances at long-term survivorship?

We also didn't know if the status of my breast cancer changed. I had a video-assisted thoracic surgery, or VATS lung biopsy, which showed the cancer was still ER- and HER2-positive. I didn't realize the VATS lung biopsy was major surgery. They went into the left lung to take out two nodules to investigate them. Because I had so much scarring and adhesions on my left lung from my spine surgery, there was a lot of bleeding. I came through and healed relatively quickly from the lung surgery. Yet the doctors and nurses did not tell me in the hospital that because of the bleeding, I had become very anemic, which caused chronic headaches. Until I found out about the anemia a month later when I was getting blood work, I worried I had brain metastases. In all, it took me about six months to recover from the anemia.

I've had multiple chemotherapies, anti-hormonal therapies, HER2 therapies, radiation therapies, a blood transfusion, and surgeries to my breast, spine, and lung. I've gone through eleven cancer drugs in the past twelve years in different doses and combinations. It's been an adventure. I'm on Kadcyla now since 2013. The first scan showed significant tumor size reduction after treatment. All the following scans have shown a consistent yet slow rate of growth in my existing lung tumors, but not enough to warrant a change in therapy yet.

I have been in a committed relationship since 2007. I met my boyfriend three months after my lung metastases diagnosis. In May 2013, we were shocked yet delighted to learn I was pregnant. I didn't think it could happen because of all my years and number of treatments and my age. I stopped treatments for three weeks after discovering I was pregnant to figure out what to do. We discussed my situation with my oncologist, and I further consulted with a medical geneticist, a gynecologist, a fetal medicine specialist specializing in cancer patients, a medical intuitive, a rabbi, and a chaplain. Both my oncologist and my gynecologist recommended I not continue with the pregnancy because all my treatments were highly toxic to embryos and fetuses, especially during the first trimester. In addition, I would also have to stop all cancer treatments for the first trimester and that was very dangerous. The cancer could spread quickly in my body and become life threatening fast. I wanted the baby but the risks to my health and life and to the healthy development and life of the fetus were very great. With an ultrasound in my sixth week, I discovered I had a miscarriage.

It was a very difficult time, but I think the pregnancy made us realize how much we really meant to each other. My partner had little experience with major illness in his family when we met, but he's been with me every step of the way. After ten days of dating, he came with me to treatment. And he was there for my lung surgery, every major oncology appointment, and all of my medical issues, side effects, and emotional rollercoaster rides thereafter. He has had a good influence on me, helping me lead a healthier lifestyle and mindset.

Whenever I talk with single women going through breast cancer, even metastatic breast cancer, I tell them dating and a loving relationship are very possible and real. You don't have to think because you have a chronic illness that no one will be interested in you, or that you don't want to burden anyone with your issues, medical or otherwise.

A relationship means they want to be there. I met my partner at a difficult time for me. I was just diagnosed with new metastases to my lungs and about to start a new course of treatment. We have the predictable ups and downs of any relationship. We've gone through a lot, individually and together.

I correlate optimism with trying to do your best to live a good life. I believe that finding the right mind and body approach can lead to living long and well. It doesn't mean I'm happy all the time and always doing the right thing. I get depressed at times. When I get down, I start eating junk, and my mind and self-talk go to places that are probably not the healthiest. I have periods of low energy, not taking great care of myself, or isolating myself from people.

I think it's important to allow yourself to feel your emotions ... with the caveat that long-term depression is not healthy. My self-criticism gets in the way of making each moment count. It helps to speak up and share your feelings, either with a counselor or a support group or a supportive, nurturing person in your life. I think sometimes having metastatic cancer creates pressure on us to live the perfect life. People might say, "Because you have cancer, it's more critical for you to take good care of yourself and have a good mental attitude than for someone without cancer." I don't see the difference. I am dealing with cancer, but cancer is not who I am. I have the same struggles as everyone else.

Sometimes when I'm down, I wonder if I'm wasting my life away with bad habits instead of taking advantage of every moment, especially since I don't know how limited my time on this earth is. Some of my past treatments, particularly the estrogen suppression treatments, sent me into a deep depression. I decided to go on antidepressants and go to therapy. I thought, *I don't want to live in this mindset.*

I'm much better at catching myself now with supportive self-talk, but it required a lot of help through counseling and support groups. I "check in" and say to myself, "This won't last forever. It has gotten better in the past and it will get better again. Let's find a way to make it better." Sometimes it's just taking a shower or getting dressed and getting off the sofa. Other times, I'll pass up French fries and choose something healthy like a salad. I don't feel guilty that I'm not always cooking the healthiest things or juicing and eating everything organic. I do the best I can for today, and work as much as possible on maintaining a healthy mind and body for the long-term.

Just a week ago I ate a fried fish sandwich and French fries I bought at a place down the street. I felt guilty about it, but finally after four days that urge left me, and I got back to eating healthier and exercising. Being active and eating well made me feel better mentally and physically. I realize that for a few days, I may not be as vigilant as usual but I don't have to murder myself for it.

People have to give themselves a break to be human. I think there's pressure that if you have cancer, you need to change your whole life around. But everyone has their own capabilities, and you can't force one form of solution or technique on someone. Everybody needs to find their own healthy and constructive way to a physically, emotionally, and mentally fulfilling and meaningful life and shouldn't feel they have to live up to someone else's ideal.

Because of my cancer experiences, I became a volunteer global peer counselor and advocate for breast cancer patients and their families. It mixed my two interests: biology of cancer and being social. When I worked in a lab, I got tired of taking care of cells in Petri dishes. This way I can learn the biology of cancer and talk to peers at the same time. I can help guide people dealing with breast cancer from diagnosis to recovery and to find resources.

I felt alone and lost when I was first diagnosed so I work hard to share with others that they don't have to feel this way. When I do public speaking, I'll tell audiences not to blame themselves for their cancer. You didn't give yourself cancer from your lifestyle, stress, or thought processes. If thousands of researchers don't know the cause of breast cancer, how would you know what causes it?

It's very important to me that survivors know that we are all here for each other as peers and supporters and watching each other's backs. No one has to feel like they're going to fall off an emotional cliff from this disease. None of us have to deal with it alone.

I want to ensure we have the best and most comprehensive support, guidance, and resources we all deserve . . . not just to survive, but to enduringly thrive. Knowing I'm helping my community of peers and receiving their support in return brings more meaning to this crazy and unexpected ride.

There is so much more to this ongoing story than even what is written here. It continues to be shaped as we firmly insist upon and strive for full and healthy lives.

Lessons Learned

- We can accept ourselves and the fact that we're not perfect and can't always act perfectly. Just try to be healthier in mind and body and make life in general better for yourself and others.
- Feeling down sometimes is normal, but long-term depression can be harmful. Seek professional help and/or share with people who you trust and can help and learn constructive and healthy ways you can lift yourself up. Think of something you can do today that will make you feel satisfied and happy.
- There is a lot of pressure to be independent in our society, but community support and help is important for long-term cancer recovery. Having support, in whatever forms to best improve your life, is essential.

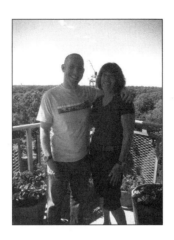

Going with the Flow

Flo Singer
Raleigh, NC
Age 66
Diagnosed with stage IV rectal cancer in 2002 and stage II lung
cancer in 2012

I was the middle child in between two boys. My parents were eastern European and Jewish. For some people in this culture, boys are much more valuable than girls. That's how I felt growing up, even though I did very well in school and was recognized for it.

My mother was a narcissist. I am grateful to her because her rejection of me taught me not to be like her. I thought I got over my anger about how my mother treated me as a child and even as an adult, but true forgiveness is a hard thing to do. I thought I worked it out with therapy. It took having cancer for it to hit me that I was holding in all this anger.

In the winter of 2001, I went to my OB/GYN for my yearly checkup. He told me I was five years overdue for a colonoscopy and referred me to a proctologist. The proctologist wouldn't make eye contact, which is really important in this type of relationship, so I didn't come back.

Four or five months later in March, I was watching Katie Couric on TV talking about colon cancer. So I called my nurse practitioner who gave me the name of a gastroenterologist who I went to see. I just went in to get the colonoscopy and figured that would be that. I had no symptoms; I was fine. I just went because it was time to go.

I was ready to leave the office and the nurse said, "No, go into his office; he wants to talk with you." He walked in and without any preliminaries, said, "Flo, I'm really sorry but you have rectal cancer."

I was floored and still a little dizzy from anesthesia. Once I was more conscious, I felt like somebody shot me between the eyes. If you touched me, you would knock me out of the chair. Sometimes people play the game, "How do you think you're going to die?" I always said, "Old age." I never thought I would get cancer.

I said, "At least we caught it early," not realizing that if he could see it with his naked eye, it was advanced. He said, "No. I've taken the liberty of making an appointment for you with a surgeon."

I called my son Michael and he asked, "How did it go?" And I said, "Not so well." He said, "I'll be right over." That was it; he went with me to my surgeon.

I had no symptoms—no pain, discomfort, or bleeding. I look back and maybe I saw some mucus in the bowl in the bathroom, but I didn't think it was anything. I was going through menopause; there were so many changes in my body that I attributed it to that.

The surgeon told me that the bad thing about colon cancer is that there are no symptoms. That's why getting a colonoscopy is so important. If you have precancerous polyps, it can be fixed right during the colonoscopy.

When I asked him about my odds, he told me I had 20 percent chance of survival. That's when I got scared. He told me, "But odds don't mean anything. It all depends on how you respond to treatment."

The tumor was inside my rectum. It was so large, it had already penetrated the intestinal wall. And they found it was already in my lymph nodes. He said they got everything with the surgery.

It was a real big shock initially. I didn't share my prognosis with anyone for about six weeks except for my children and my mother because it took me those six weeks to process the information. I had to integrate what I spiritually believed with the reality of my condition.

I felt quite relieved once I accepted the fact that I had such advanced cancer. My body might die, but I believed I would always be here because of the immortality of the soul. I knew treatment would cure me or death would. It was a deliberate choice to look at it that way. I also felt that I wanted to set an example for my adult children that death is just part of the life cycle.

I'm a Jewish Buddhist, a "Jewbu," so I believe in reincarnation. They have done research that the difference between a person's weight when they are alive and dead is about 8 milligrams. I believe the difference is the essence of who you are. Some people call it the soul.

Even if it's not, the energy that was giving off the electrical charge (EKG or EEG) is no longer there. Energy cannot be destroyed, it can change form. To me, that is scientific proof that there is a soul or essence of who you are that leaves the body after death.

I look at death as a new adventure, not as the ending. So I'm not afraid to die. As soon as I came to this realization during the first six weeks, I was okay with whatever was going to happen. Because I knew who I am. Flosey, the nutty girl that I am, is going to be around, maybe somewhere in another dimension. The more I thought about it, the stronger my belief and optimism became.

At that time, they did chemo a little differently than they do now. I had a port inserted and was getting 5-FU and Leucovorin, 24/7, six days a week for six weeks straight. I developed neuropathy in my feet and I lost about four teeth.

In addition to that, every day in the morning when I was going to work as a hair stylist, I went in to get radiation. I had four passes of radiation per day, five days a week for six weeks straight. It was a horror. After the first week, I couldn't sit, so I had to have friends drive me to work. I still could stand and lay down, but internally, I was burned beyond belief. It was exceptionally painful until they got me on morphine pills.

Michael, who was thirty at the time, lived in the next town over, and my daughter Stephanie, twenty-six, was in Chicago at the time. They were extremely supportive to say the least, and so were my friends. Whenever I had to go to the doctor, Michael would come with me. He insisted on that. I was fine during the week but during the weekends, I spent most of the time in the emergency room.

People don't want to talk about colorectal cancer because of the part of the body involved. It is a tough thing. I talked with my clients about it as I was cutting their hair. Several of them, who never had colonoscopies, went to get one because of my story. Three of them had precancerous polyps.

Some days, my clients would go to the pharmacy or grocery shopping with me. I don't usually mix business with pleasure and I always found if you got too close, especially as a hair stylist, a barrier was broken. But I accepted their help. I was amazed at the love that was coming from them.

People would say to me, "Do you ever think, 'why me?'" And my answer was, "Why not me?" I believed things happened, not for a reason, but for a purpose. I believed in my soul that cancer was a disease of anger. I thought that I had resolved a number of my anger issues, but realized I didn't. Louise Hay talks about holding things in. There were issues involving my mother, and I realized I needed to let go. I used humor a lot to help me cope with my situation. I've always used humor even as a kid because I found if people were smiling they couldn't bite you.

After I finished chemo and radiation, I had a month's rest before surgery. My surgeon was a very formal kind of guy. During my second visit with him, we went into the examining room with his nurse. I saw on his tray of instruments something that looked like a speculum, but this thing was really huge. I said, "Hey doc, you plan on using that on me?" I was really frightened. And he answered, "Miss Singer, don't tell me you're a scaredy cat."

I replied, "Listen, normally a guy has to take me to a really good dinner and movie before I let him do anything like that!" He looked at me, "Miss Singer, I'm a married man!" I laughed, "Doc, it was just a joke!" But I admitted I was scared.

He reassured me by saying, "I'll be as gentle as I can." So I said, "I'll tell you what, since we're going to be so up close and personal, you can call me Flo and I can call you Eric."

After that, I could drop trow in a heartbeat. There's no bit of modesty left in me. He loosened up after that and we'd joke all the time. We have a great relationship.

I had the same type of relationship with my radiation oncologist. Just days after surgery, he was examining me and asked, "Does this hurt?"

I answered, "You mean other than the fact you have a finger up my butt?" I thought it was kind of funny. He started laughing and said, "I've been doing this for twenty-five years and no one has said that to me."

I replied, "Don't you think it's about time?" He said, "I think I'm going to enjoy being your doctor, Flo."

But I wasn't always joking with my doctors. My belief is that the doctors aren't doing me any favors. I'm paying them; I hired them. If they no longer serve their purpose, I'll move on to another doctor. There are lots of other doctors out there.

During my surgery, they took out about eighteen inches of my colon. My surgeon was wonderful. I asked him how many of his patients died of rectal cancer. He said to me, "I never had a patient who died of rectal cancer, and you're not going to be my first."

I can't tell you the kind of relief, inspiration, and faith I had because of what he said and his positive attitude! I always try to have positive people around me.

I was frightened because I didn't want to have a colostomy bag. Before I went into surgery, he asked me, "If it's a choice between dying and having a colostomy, what do you want?" Of course, we know the answer to that. "If I have to do colostomy, I'll try to reverse it in six months."

I didn't need a colostomy, but I was in the hospital for a week. Again, I realized I'd have to be my own advocate. I was in a lot of pain and developed a rash, infection, and fever from the radiation, which they couldn't eliminate. At one point, a nurse came in to examine me, and she wasn't wearing gloves. I said to her, "You have to wash your hands and put on a pair of gloves if you're going to examine me."

She asked, "Oh, is that important to you?" I said that it was. She was an oncology nurse; don't you think she'd realize her patients have compromised immune systems?

Once a doctor came in and took a pair of gloves. I said, "No, if you want to examine me, you have to wash your hands and then put on a pair of gloves." He looked at me and I continued, "Unless you can guarantee that the doorknob is sterile, you're not getting near me." He replied, "You're right, Flo." And I said that I appreciated it.

I was always very nice, but I was the first priority, not their feelings. After doing a lot of research online, I found out that over one hundred thousand people die of staph infections in hospitals for this very reason. I always made sure nurses used sanitizer before doing anything. I became crazy that way, but I never had a staph infection.

The first three days I couldn't eat anything. I had tubes in every orifice of my body. My daughter and her fiancé stayed with me for the first two weeks after surgery. I couldn't stand up by myself. I had to learn to walk all over again and wear diapers because I couldn't make it to the bathroom in time. But my kids were there for me, which was a really big to-do.

I would find myself at times breaking out sobbing for no reason. About a month after surgery, I went to the dentist and when he leaned the chair back, all of a sudden I started crying. He was shocked because

I presented such a strong front. He just held me and said, "You've been through so much, honey, this is probably scaring you. We can take care of this in two weeks."

I woke up every day, even when I was going through treatment, and gave myself permission to have a five-minute pity party before my morning shower. Then I'd say, "Okay, it's show time!" I put on this mask and tried to "fake it until I make it." Despite how I felt, I really believed I'd be alright.

Every night when I'd take a bath, I would visualize that I was healthy and the healthy cells were getting rid of cancer cells. I saw myself as a vibrant woman doing everything I wanted to do.

I kept a journal every single day. I fully believe you create your own reality. So I'd ask myself, *What do I want to create here?* On the first page, I'd list all the things I was grateful for. On the next page I would state, "I am" or "I have," as if everything I wanted had already taken place. Because if you say, "I want," you end up with the wanting instead of the having. I would state, "I'm in great health," even though I wasn't. I was going to put myself in great health. So what I wanted and what I created would catch up with each other. This would reinforce within me all the things I really believed. At times it was hard, but usually I would choose to make it a good day. Each day, I would consciously decide that was the day something wonderful would happen.

These practices continued to help me even when surgery and treatment was over. For years I had side effects. Seven years after my treatment, I lost all my top teeth and had to get implants. It also did damage to my digestive system.

I used to call my surgeon about my bathroom habits. I'd tell him, "I feel like a kid talking to my daddy about her bowel movements." He said, "That's all right. We assaulted your body with radiation and chemo because you had such an advanced case. Your intestines are so thinned out that they are never going to react the way they used to to it."

I could live with that, but I didn't know how true it was. For three years, I took two Imodiums before each meal, and if I went out at night,

81

I'd take another two. I always had a change of clothing in the car. Even to this day, I may be in the middle of a conversation and I'll have to say, "Hold that thought," and run to the bathroom. It's something I have learned is just part of the new me.

My gastroenterologist calls me his miracle patient because the odds were against me getting through this. I think that by believing that I'd be cured, laughing a lot, creating my own well-being—along with good treatments—helped me survive. Another important factor was the love and friendship of the people around me. I had everybody praying for me. I told one friend who's a Muslim, "You better pray to Allah for me!"

Looking back, it was a sense of relief to be alive, but there was also the fear of "Is this is what it's going to be for the rest of my life?" and "Will it come back?" I think that's part of the cancer continuum patients face, no matter what kind of cancer they have. Because I wanted to help others going through that continuum, I decided to go back to school to become a cancer coach.

There are so many issues involved with this kind of cancer. There are sexual problems and how you feel about your body image. I was cut from stem to stern and had this god-awful scar. It took me a couple of years to wake up and not think about cancer.

Cancer came to the forefront again, however, in 2012. I turned sixty-five and prior to that, I didn't have insurance. So I went on Medicare. I was having this pain in my groin. I ignored it because so many people have these types of issues after having my kind of surgery. But it got to the point that I was doubled up in pain and couldn't move. My internist couldn't figure out what it was, so I went to my oncologist, a different one than who I saw the first time. He referred me to a surgeon.

When the surgeon examined me, he said, "I don't know what's going on. You haven't had a CT scan in nine years. Let's have one."

Two days later, he said, "Great news, there's no cancer in your intestines, but we found a mass in your lung." I asked if this was the old cancer or a new one. He said, after ten years, it was a new cancer. He ordered a PET scan, which confirmed it.

It blew me away; I was totally unprepared for it. It was a bigger shock than the first time. The following week I went into surgery to have a third of my lung removed.

It was non–small cell carcinoma, which is the best kind of lung cancer to get. It was early, stage II, not in the lymph nodes. My oncologist said that I was really lucky to have pain, which was unusual for this type of cancer. He told me, "Had you not come in for it, by the time you would have felt something in your lung, you'd be too far gone to do anything about it."

I did well with the surgery, but the chemo was devastating. Michael came in from New York when I had the surgery, and Stephanie came in from LA when I had chemo a month later. I only had four treatments but I was totally wrecked. I was nauseous, lost my hair, and had no strength. I couldn't move from the couch. It was a metal-based chemo, which wreaks havoc on your body. I totally hadn't expected it; it was totally out of left field, and I dropped out of life for a while.

The fear of dying wasn't there, but I knew I would have to become a new me again. I was ten years older than I was when I had rectal cancer and I didn't know if I'd have the strength to do it. I was depressed, so I went on antidepressants, which helped, but I had to really work to get my mind in a good place and reconcile having cancer again.

I thought, *I survived* stage *IV rectal cancer, and now this? Give me a break!* I told Michael, "I'm an organ donor, but I planned on doing it when I was dead, not living."

I had to grow my lung capacity back and start walking. It was like starting from square one again. I felt like the universe had hit me over the head with a two-by-four.

Family and friends were so supportive. They would say, "Take all the time you need. You are your first priority, not your clients. You need to get yourself straight." I called up another cancer coach to get coaching.

It took over a year to do the emotional work and insert myself back into living, but it was worth it.

I read once that you teach what you have to learn the most. I feel I can understand what people are going through physically, emotionally, and spiritually. That's why I became a coach. I feel I'm really reinforcing to my clients and myself something I really believe. I'm saying, "Don't do as I say but as I do." By helping clients, I'm helping myself.

It's like having a glass of water. When it's empty you can't share it with anybody; when it's full—meaning you're in a good place—you can take that and share it. I don't give my clients the answers; I just give them questions and they come up with their own answers.

Everybody knows their own truth. They have to get down to the basics of what they believe. Just because they have cancer, doesn't mean they *are* cancer. They have a right to a good, healthy life for as long or a short as it is. I have no guarantees. We're all going to die—it's how we live that matters.

I'm doing great today. Michael and his wife decided to move to Tokyo. En route, they found out she was pregnant again. They had tried for years, so it was exciting. When the baby was two months old, I flew out to see my grandson. It gave me something to live for. I love being a grandma. Seeing my children raise their children makes my heart swell.

No matter what's going to happen, I've decided I'm going to live in the moment and enjoy what I have right now. If I worry about things, I'm still going to end up in the same place anyway. Worrying is just a waste of good energy. I wake up in the morning and decide what's going to happen today. Today, I chose again to have a good day.

Lessons Learned

- You can write the ending of your story. It's what you choose to believe that will guide your life. It's not your dying; it's your living that's important.
- Surround yourself with people who are going to support whatever you decide to do. You're the only one who knows what's right for you. Sometimes you need help finding out what that is—whether it's therapy, a coach, or journaling—but it's important.
- We can choose every day how we live life. Choose happiness over sadness. Choose optimism over pessimism. Choose love instead of fear.

You can learn more about Flo and contact her at www.flowinglifecoaching.com.

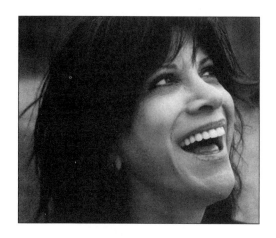

A Stage Is for Tap Dancing

GLENINE GREGORY-RYAN
Wurtsboro, NY
Age 58
Diagnosed with Hodgkin Disease in 1977 and stage IV meta-plastic carcinoma (a rare form of breast cancer) in 2001

As I look back, I choose to only remember the good. I was born an only child to Italian parents in Newburg, NY, a beautiful little city along the Hudson. We lived in my grandmother's apartment building. My aunt lived upstairs, my grandmother on the middle floor, my mother's cousin on the top floor, and we were in the basement apartment. There was always Italian flurry, as I used to call it. The house always smelled wonderful from cooking, and there was lots of tradition. We played stickball in the streets and ate ice pops in the summer. When I got older, we moved to the suburbs. My parents divorced when I was thirteen.

During my freshman year of college, I met a rock musician who was much older than me. I fell in love and left college to marry him. My first daughter, Lauren, is from that marriage.

When Lauren was one, I dropped a tremendous amount of weight but thought it was from running around with a baby. I developed tumors in my neck, which doctors originally thought was an infection, but decided to do a biopsy. The first biopsy came back negative because they didn't get enough of the tumor. Everyone was overjoyed, but meanwhile, more tumors were popping up. Finally, they did a biopsy of two whole glands and were able to see the cells and determined I had Hodgkin's lymphoma. By that time, I had twenty-seven tumors in the neck and six in the chest.

I went on chemotherapy for nine months. My last chemotherapy was on my twenty-second birthday. I also had upper mantel radiation, which set me up with some nasty breast cancer twenty-five years later. Back then, they only had Compazine for nausea, and it wasn't enough, so I was sick for about forty-eight hours straight after chemo. I remember going home one day through the George Washington Bridge and vomiting into an airplane sick bag.

I took it in stride. I had a baby and husband to live for, and I was planning to go back to school to be a nurse. I thought, "Let's just get through this." I didn't dwell on it. At the time, Hodgkin's was just starting to be curable. I always looked forward—it's my personality. It was a matter of survival; I had to raise my daughter, and there's no way I was leaving.

The treatment worked, and I was cancer-free . . . until a few days before Thanksgiving in 2001. I found a lump while doing a breast self-exam. It was very pronounced and hard. I went to a gynecologist friend who got me right in and sent me to get a mammogram. They saw a solid, white mass that was the size of a quarter and perfectly round. At first they thought it was a fibroadenoma (a benign lump), but I had a biopsy and variety of tests done that confirmed it was breast cancer.

They thought I was stage II for about four days, but upon having a PET scan, they found a metastasis in my lung. I found a wonderful doctor at Sloan Kettering who excised the tumor. After the surgery, she told me I had stage IV metaplastic carcinoma, a very rare and aggressive form of breast cancer. At the time, it represented only .01 percent of breast cancer cases. She told me, "You have probably six months to live."

I thought about a Bible story of the man who lay by the pool at Bethesda for thirty years. Once a year, the angel came and cured whoever got to the water first. But he was on a mat; he couldn't move his legs. Jesus came by and the man said, "Jesus, help me!" And Jesus said, "Take your mat and go home; you are healed," and he did.

I remember saying to myself, "Self, take your mat and go home." I rang the nurse and asked her to get a resident to remove my chest tubes because I was leaving. Everyone told me I couldn't do that, but I convinced them to remove the chest tubes. I was home for Christmas, and on December 26, I went looking for an oncologist who was going to treat me. I couldn't just sit back and let this engulf me.

I found I had to defend myself for not thinking I was going to die. A stage is something to tap dance on. I'm not a stage. The statistics were five to six years old and I wasn't buying it. People were telling me to get my affairs in order; oncologists told me they didn't want to treat me. One said, "If we give you chemotherapy, it's only going to come back. It's that aggressive."

I was a nurse from '78 to '92, and I think it made me more of a squeaky wheel to get things done. I knew doctors were not God, and they put their pants on the way we all did. Just because one highly esteemed doctor told me I was going to die, it didn't make it true. Who the hell are you? Do you see an expiration tag on my toe? That's how I always carried it through.

I found a wonderful oncologist in New Jersey at a progressive cancer center and brought all my pathology slides to him. He looked at them and asked me, "What do you want to do?" Through tears I said, "I want to fight like hell. I want you to hit me with everything you've got!"

I asked him how many metaplastic carcinoma cases he had seen. He only saw one, but he called friends at Dana Farber and MD Anderson who had a protocol for it. So I had a triangle of doctors working with me.

I received a huge dose of Adriamycin for three months. Zofran really controlled the nausea, but I had to keep up with it because the Adriamycin dosage was so high. Basically I was a guinea pig because there weren't many studies on metaplastic carcinoma. They just winged it. I had Neulasta, so I never had problems with blood counts.

A day after Mother's Day, I had a double mastectomy and reconstruction. After I recovered from that, I did three months of Taxotere. My PET scans ever since have shown no evidence of disease.

There were times when I had what I called "hankerings," and wanted nothing but bagels and cream cheese or chicken salad. When that was the only thing I could hold down, I ate it. I ate my vegetables, but if I wanted a piece of pumpkin pie with whipped cream, I ate it. If I wanted a martini, I drank it.

I think people don't enjoy the little things in life because they think if they eat that chocolate chip cookie their cancer is going to come roaring back. What does guilt do to your psyche? It's not the chocolate chip cookie putting the stress on you; it's the guilt.

For me, the toughest part was the exhaustion. I was about to have a double mastectomy and I remember being so exhausted I joked, "You don't have to give me any anesthetic; I'll be asleep before the lights go on."

I was very blessed to have support from my husband, family, and friends. Fortunately, we were okay financially so I didn't have to work. Did that contribute to my well-being? Absolutely! I wish everybody could have had what I had during that time.

My faith played a big role, too. After my mastectomy, I turned my life over to Jesus Christ and became born again. I read a little pamphlet that had Bible quotes about how Jesus healed the sick. It was so nurturing and comforting that I literally wore the book out. I embraced the fact that God didn't give me cancer—he allowed it and gave me a way to get through it.

Every day, someone would call from church to ask how I was doing. They'd say, "We're praying for you and by the way, I left you a casserole." Or somebody would say, "You're a warrior; you can do this." If I felt a little shaky, I knew I could call somebody.

Once, I was having a really bad day and saw a card from a cancer organization that had a number you could call to speak to a peer. I called and a woman named Joy answered. I told her my story, and she said, "Are you sitting down? I was you sixteen years ago in the early '80s." She had the same kind of cancer. It was in her lungs, and the doctor gave her three months. She got all the chemo she could get and outlived her oncologist.

Then she told me, "I don't normally answer the phones. This is amazing! I just do secretarial work and public relations. The fact I went past this ringing phone and picked it up and we shared our stories, there's got to be a higher authority."

Would I want to go through cancer again? No. But what an amazing journey to see how much you can handle with support and your faith! Some people feel isolated, but in this day and age, no one needs to feel that way.

I believe you give and you get back. I survived cancer twice; who gets a second chance? I've been given it, so I have to turn it around and make something positive out of it. If I can lift up someone for ten seconds, that's ten seconds they don't feel the weight of the world. When I'm speaking with patients who have this type of diagnosis, I tell them, "I'm no different than you are. You're still breathing. It's today; do what you can so you can be here tomorrow."

Maybe I have a Pollyanna attitude and see the glass as half full. Maybe I don't spend time on "what ifs." If that's denial, it's been working for me for twelve years. I don't deny that cancer kills, but I never felt it was in the cards for me to die.

For me, there wasn't a lot of "I can't do this" because I had to do it. I just didn't give death an option. I had three children and was newly remarried when I received my stage IV diagnosis. Cancer wasn't taking me when I was twenty-one and it wasn't taking me when I was forty-six. I was always a goal achiever, but it wasn't until I had cancer that I knew it was do or die.

Ten years into my marriage, my husband left me, but I have to thank him for being my right arm. Without him, I don't know what I would have done. Sometimes that's what gets me through when I get angry. All of a sudden I'm single and dating. I never tell guys about my cancer until the third date. I learned to get to know them first before lowering the boom, but eventually they have to know. Some guys think if you're stage IV, you're on death's door. I've had some who said they couldn't handle it, which is fine. But I've had some nice relationships. I'm in a great one now.

I went to my last oncologist checkup in April 2013. He said, "I don't want to keep scanning you. You have had enough to light up New York City. I'm going to let you go, but before I do, I want you to read the first page of your chart." I read, "Progression will be noted and likelihood of survival is less than one year." I went to the last page, where he wrote, "Dismissed" in red marker with a big smiley face.

I just moved to upstate New York and am getting ready to buy a new home. I'm going to do what I do best—live. I have a granddaughter, Piper, who's five. My boyfriend and I love to hike, go shopping, and go to movies. Life is grand. The divorce was hard, even worse than the cancer, but life is good again. I wish that for everyone. My biggest wish, however, is that they find a cure and a scientist in a lab somewhere who will say, "Eureka, we did it!"

Lessons Learned

- See cancer as the rearview mirror in your car. You have to look at it from time to time, but you have to use the windshield that's in front of you (your life).
- Never give up. I'm not putting down someone who does, but that's not in my makeup. I'm going to go out kicking and screaming.
- Treat yourself. When you're first diagnosed with stage IV and you're reading statistics, you could think, "Why would I buy that nice sweater and only get five years' wear out of it?" Go buy it and plan on being around to wear it!

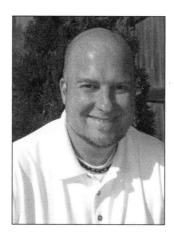

The Power of Positivity

GREG CANTWELL
Coralville, IA
Age 40
Diagnosed in 2004 with stage IV glioblastoma multiforme (most aggressive form of brain cancer)

We lived in West Germany when I was a child. There was still an East and West Germany then. It wouldn't be unheard of to see tanks going down the road.

My father was the principal of the American International School of Dusseldorf. One night, the school was bombed by the Baader Meinhof gang, Irish Republic Army, and the Red Brigade. These groups had gang members in different prisons throughout West Germany and Europe, and they wanted them to be housed in one location. Because the bombing happened during the night, nobody was hurt, but I remember my dad taking me to school the next day and bringing me right back home. Many buildings were damaged by the blast and smoke. It was very traumatic;

I couldn't believe something like that would happen at my school, much less a school my father ran.

About twenty years later, I had another bomb dropped on me. I was thirty, married, and had a son, Joseph, who was nine months old. I had just flown in from Hawaii to Minnesota to start a new job in the airline industry. My (now ex) wife and Joseph were already there waiting for me at the hotel. That night, I had a grand mal seizure. She later told me I woke her up because I couldn't breathe and sounded like a dying cow trying to gasp for air. She called 911, and I remember sitting at the end of the bed as the paramedics were asking me questions. It was extremely frustrating because I knew the answers to the questions, but I couldn't say them.

I consider it a miracle I survived the seizure. Prior to moving to Hawaii, I worked in Alaska for two weeks. Neither Hawaii nor Alaska, in my opinion, has great health care. The night before, I was alone in my apartment in Hawaii, since my wife and Joseph were already in Minnesota finishing up the packing. If I would have had the seizure that night in the apartment by myself, I would have been dead. I believe somebody upstairs was looking after me and waited until the last possible moment for the seizure—when I was in a state with good health care and had someone there to help me.

I don't remember much of what transpired. They did an MRI and CT scan when I got to the hospital and told me they needed to call in a neurologist from his home. I was thinking to myself, "Why are they doing this?"

The neurologist came in that night and told me that I had a mass in my head and needed to have a biopsy, which they scheduled three days later. When the results came back, the neurosurgeon and neuro-oncologist told me I had stage IV glioblastoma multiforme (GBM—the most rare and aggressive form of primary brain cancer), and my chances of living more than a year were very slim.

At first I thought, *How could this happen to me? I've led a good life, and I always tried to help people.* The feeling sorry for myself lasted twenty-four to forty-eight hours; then I thought, *Okay, this is what it is, so there's nothing I can do right now to turn back the clock. I'm going to do whatever I can to give me the best chance at surviving and beating this.*

I wanted to make sure I would be here to see Joseph graduate from high school, have girlfriends, play sports, go to college, and get married. He was my driving force.

My diagnosis was quite a shock to me, but looking back at it, I had two or three migraines a year and had gone to see doctors about it. Not once did they do a CT or MRI. They just kept prescribing drugs to deal with the effects of the migraine. In hindsight, I had all the symptoms of a brain tumor: blurry vision, equilibrium problems, vomiting, difficulties with talking, and numbness that started with my fingers and went all the way up my arms. My doctors just dismissed them as migraine symptoms.

The neuro-oncologist gave me three treatment options. I had time to research them and call a couple of friends who were neuro-oncologists and surgeons for their opinions. I chose the most aggressive form of treatment, which included having Gliadel Wafers placed into the resected tumor site to provide direct chemotherapy to the leftover cancer cells. After recovery from surgery, radiation, and six weeks of Temodar, I began carboplatin, using an intra-arterial method that delivers high-dose chemotherapy through the artery in the groin to the brain. A catheter is used, which is threaded up into the brain where the medication is released. It required twelve months of treatment and for me to be in a hospital during treatments once a month. I didn't know the side effects of the five chemo drugs I would be taking, but I chose it because it gave me the best chance of long-term survival.

I was fortunate I didn't have to work through treatment and still had insurance coverage. I did go to work the day after I had my grand mal seizure. It was my first day on the job and I let them know what was happening. They told me I could work that day, so I could get benefits and be kept on their insurance. I had to go on COBRA, but that was a godsend because I had my insurance for thirty days from my previous job. Between the two insurance policies, I was covered 100 percent for my surgery and the first month of treatment.

Even though they didn't know me, human resources set it up so people could donate their vacation time, and I'd get a paycheck at the person's pay rate. That helped pay toward medical bills and COBRA payments.

I'm also so lucky I have such a close and supportive family. They all flew in to make sure they would be here for me because none of us knew how long I had. My brother Chris, who's next oldest to me, actually moved his entire family from Virginia to Minnesota so they were available to support and take care of me.

I was very nauseous and fatigued from the treatments. They gave me medication for the nausea, but I had to take naps two or three times a day due to fatigue. I could have stayed in bed all day, but I knew I had to move around to avoid blood clots and live as normal a life as possible. I got out as much as I could, but took into account to listen to my body when it was time to relax.

Every time I went for a treatment, I knew I could potentially die. The cancer was so aggressive, and the chance of me having a stroke or a blood clot during treatment was very real.

I have always been a positive, strong person, and that's how I confronted this. I wanted to continue my life as normally as possible. I remember I had staples in my head after surgery and went to the Mall of America with the family. People stared at me, but who cares?

When I went into the hospital for my treatments, I made sure I was able to smile and have a sense of humor and that nurses and everyone else knew my personality. It was as important to me to laugh as it was for me to get the nurses to laugh and get their minds off of the hard situations they dealt with working on the cancer floor. People ask me if I got depressed; I don't know what depression feels like. I just always wanted to make people laugh, not worry, and make it through.

The treatments were working and eventually I received the words, "Your MRIs are stable; there's no sign of progression." I haven't had any recurrences, but I don't use the word, "remission." There are always cancer cells, and I know I could be fine today, and the tumor could be back tomorrow. It grows that fast.

But going through this, I never had the opportunity to talk to another brain cancer survivor, much less one with GBM. I didn't know anybody who had a brain tumor and neither did my friends and family. My doctors' hands were tied due to the Privacy Act. I tried to go to a support group but that brought my morale down and I wanted to remain strong, positive, and full of hope.

In 2007, I started a website, *www.survivorandcaregiver.com*, to see who else was out there. I was several years out from my treatment and wanted to give back. I knew how invaluable having someone to talk with would have been to me. The only person who truly knows what you're going through, even though you react differently to treatments, is a person who's been there before. I got forty thousand hits from all over the world in the first two months. People in all stages of their diagnosis contacted me. To this day, I still receive emails from that site requesting help. I will never take that site down.

In 2012, I started my nonprofit, *www.gregsmission.org*, which provides support, hope, education, current resources, and awareness to patients with brain tumors, especially GBM, through phone, email, Skype, and personal visits. I will even go to their doctors' appointments with them if requested. I've been traveling around the country, speaking at cancer centers, hospitals, and pharmaceutical companies. I volunteer at all the major cancer centers in the United States for the Children's Brain Tumor Foundation, and as a brain cancer mentor for Imerman Angels. MD Anderson and Cleveland Clinic also refer their brain tumor patients to me to mentor.

I work part-time at University of Iowa now, but I still don't have enough time to help all the people who contact me. It would make me so happy to have other brain cancer survivors come on board to help provide hope. I have mentored over 760 brain cancer patients and survivors. A lot of people I mentor have passed away, unfortunately, but there are hundreds of people who are living right now with a brain tumor who require support, and that number grows daily. I also help their families and caregivers. I believe it's my calling. It's why I survived.

I know I'm one of the fortunate ones. I had a proactive doctor (which is key) who wanted to do everything he could up front. He did this not only because he knew how serious it was, but because I was young and in good physical condition. So he knew I would be able to handle the "cocktail" of chemotherapies I would be receiving. And he's a neuro-oncologist, so he knows all about the brain.

I'm a very huge proponent of doctors being up-front with patients, telling them all treatments that are available, and their benefits and risks. There are very few hospitals and doctors in the United States that do intra-arterial chemotherapy using carboplatin. I'm told that most don't do it because of how invasive it is and its risk of stroke. I tell people I mentor, "It's not the doctor's choice. It's your life; do you want the chance of long-term survival? You make the decision."

That goes for the Gliadel Wafer, too. I hear from doctors, "Well it's an old treatment, and there is no data to show it works." That's their opinion; it's your decision, and your doctor should give you all the options without letting their opinion get in the way. I believe when a patient chooses their treatment, they take ownership of that choice, which in turn will hopefully create less worry and more hope.

About 97 percent of doctors are reactive, meaning they go with the standard of care and wait to see if it comes back. That's because with GBM, textbooks say there's a 100 percent chance it's going to come back. I don't believe the textbooks or statistics. I'm ten years out now and that's proof that they're wrong!

They're treating the diagnosis, not the patient, and it should be the other way around. They need to look at the person's attitude, health, and age, and if they believe they're strong enough, offer a more aggressive treatment.

On the other hand, I don't think doctors should tell patients the statistics because every person is unique. Why would you say only 5 percent of the people live over eighteen to twenty-four months? You could be talking to one of those people who are in the 5 percent. If you tell them that, they're going to get depressed and their immune system's going to suffer. It's not putting the person in the right frame of mind to want to fight.

I believe positivity and faith are as important as medical treatment. If people are depressed, I suggest watching a comedy movie. Just doing something small like laughing, smiling, or sitting in the sun increases your immune system. I try to make sure people know there is hope. Most patients who I talk to are depressed. I can hear it in their voices. I don't sugarcoat anything; I just tell them if I believed that those statistics applied to me, I wouldn't be here talking to them today.

I couldn't have accomplished what I'm doing with brain cancer survivors without the support of my wife Lisa, who I married in 2009. She believes in me, can see how passionate I am about what I do, and understands that to have a survivor to talk to is invaluable. Lisa also has a life threatening illness—cystic fibrosis, as well as diabetes. She had a liver transplant in 2009 and is one of the strongest people I know. She works full-time and supports my mission 100 percent.

Joseph is eleven now. He's very energetic and full of questions. We just want to live life to its fullest, create memories for him, and make sure our dreams come true. I still have flight benefits from my airline job, so we've been to Europe, Thailand, and Australia and plan to continue to see the world and help people along the way.

People ask me if I'm worried about the cancer coming back. I answer that it's out of my control. There is no sense worrying about it. If it does I will deal with it at that time. I can do everything I can to get the next best treatment. But there's nothing I can do right now to prevent it. Only the guy upstairs knows when and if that will happen.

We don't take life for granted anymore. It's a whole different perspective. I tell survivors, "You have a serious disease, but you have the opportunity to make sure you say I love you to your spouse and hug your family every day. People die in car accidents and they don't have that opportunity." I tell Lisa I love her every day when I drop her off at work and at night before I go to sleep . . . because if I don't come back, at least I was able to say those last words.

I've learned a lot since cancer exploded into my life. I can accept the realities of my aggressive disease while doing everything in my power to live life to its fullest and with no regrets. And I can use what I've learned to help others. Life is uncertain, but one thing I do know: Your attitude can make all the difference.

Lessons Learned

- Don't take life for granted or put things off. It's not about having the next best TV or car to show up your neighbor, or making tons of money. It's about creating memories with your family, sharing special times with your friends, and just enjoying life.
- Have hope, regardless of the illnesses. It's not just about surviving cancer; it's about having a positive mental state, which I believe affects your outcome. Everybody's different, but I feel the longer you stay positive, the longer you'll live. Sure, there are people out there who are positive and still end up passing away. It's different for each individual person, but I've found this to be true for me and other people I know.
- Find the right doctors. Make sure you have a doctor who is willing to get to know you both from a physical and mental perspective. He or she should provide you with all available treatment options, informing you of the risks and benefits of each. You get to decide which to choose.
- Staying positive can be hard at times but you have to focus on what you believe your outcome will be. I am going to kick

cancer's butt. Stay strong, get rest when you need it, and call on your friends for support. To admit you need help is not a sign of weakness. You are not a statistic! You should be treated as a patient, not as a diagnosis.

For more information about Greg and his foundation, go to www.gregsmission.org.

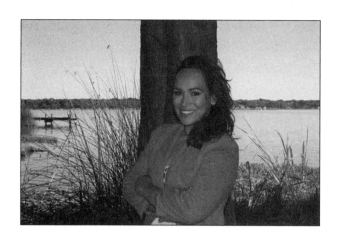

Everything Happens for a Reason

HEATHER RODRIGUEZ
Dallas, TX
Age 31
Diagnosed in 2010 with stage 3C ovarian cancer with germ
cell & epithelial tumors

I didn't have a very happy childhood. My mother had eight kids and abandoned each and every one of us at one time or another. There was physical, mental, and sexual abuse. Both my parents were mentally ill—my mother with borderline personality disorder, and my father, schizophrenia.

I was born in Arkansas, and we moved to Mexico when I was five. By the time I was six years old, I was the one raising my siblings because my mother and father were not ever around. I didn't know when I was younger that I suffered from depression, attention deficit disorder (ADD), and dyslexia.

I didn't go to school until I was ten, and we had no medical attention. My mother was a nurse, so there were a lot of things I knew.

When my brother stepped on a nail, we gave him a tetanus shot. We didn't have a bathroom, running water, or electricity. We had to use bleach to clarify water so we could drink it.

When I was sixteen, my mom decided to move back to the United States and took my sisters with her and abandoned me in a foreign country, and I've been on my own since.

I started modeling to pay for the rest of the school year. My mother then sent my two youngest sisters, Rosalinda and Imelda, who were eight and ten years younger than me, to live with me. We had no money for food. At one point I weighed only ninety pounds.

At age seventeen, my boyfriend Gregorio's mother Gina took me in like I was her daughter, along with my sisters. She was a very good example for me. Gina was very strong; she was in politics. I started to follow in her footsteps and began to learn leadership skills and a lot of other things that have served me to this day.

I went back to Arkansas, and when I was about to turn nineteen, I finished high school. When I turned twenty-five, I was given legal custody of Rosalinda and Imelda, so I couldn't finish college.

In many ways, my childhood prepared me for the challenge of my life with cancer. I look back at my life and laugh and think, "Wow, that couldn't have happened to me." When I was diagnosed with ovarian cancer, I handled it with humor. I was not surprised. I thought, of course this would happen. The craziest things happen to me. I think the overall factor in my diagnosis was so much stress in my life, and I think my body got to a point where it started shutting down. I'm just thirty-one now, and I feel like I've lived the life of a ninety-year-old.

I was misdiagnosed for nearly an entire year, at the same time my cancer was growing. It wasn't until September 22, 2010, when I was finally diagnosed with "widely spread metastatic ovarian cancer" at the age of twenty-eight. I was told I have a 10 percent survival rate.

I had typical symptoms—bloating, pain, constipation, and pain during sex. I did some research and wondered if it was ovarian cancer.

I ended up going to the ER in November 2009 because I had such terrible pain. I thought my appendix burst. They told me I had ovarian cysts, gave me a prescription for birth control pills and pain medication, and sent me home. I went to several specialists, then an internist who did blood work. The only thing it showed was that I had extremely low vitamin D levels. Then I was sent to a psychiatrist who told me I was depressed and had ADD and gave me medication for that. I was medicated for everything except for cancer.

I started feeling extremely drained—my appetite decreased and I couldn't tolerate even one drink with a friend. One day I was looking at my stomach and noticed a bump. I did a pregnancy test, and I wasn't pregnant. I told one of my friends, "I feel happy, but my body feels depressed. I feel like I'm rotting from within."

The next day we had lunch and she suggested I go to the hospital. I wasn't able to eat; the smells made me feel sick. For some reason, I knew if I went to the ER, I wasn't going to come back. I knew something was terribly wrong with me but wasn't expecting it was going to be cancer, especially such advanced cancer.

I packed a bag and went to the ER, and puked four times while they were doing scans. The doctor came back and said, "There's a mass. We can't be certain, but we think it's cancer and we have to operate now." I had to make a split-second decision at age twenty-eight.

I was so fortunate because I was close to top-notch hospitals. My two surgeons also did ovarian cancer research. In the morning I had surgery and was in for about six hours. Later, I looked through my medical records for a long time to keep track of everything. I found out they were trying to remove all the tumors and I started to hemorrhage so they had to give me blood.

They transferred me to the maternity ward, and I heard babies crying. I thought, "I'm never going to have kids!" I never wanted kids before, but didn't want my options taken away from me. I remember they woke me up, and I tried to get up and run off. The oncologist stopped me and said, "Heather you have cancer, and you're going to need chemo." That is literally how I was given the news that I had cancer, right out of my emergency surgery.

I know this sounds weird, but it was like a weight was lifted off my shoulders. I surrendered and said, "Okay, I give up; you win, whoever you are." I'm an emotional nutcase, but then I wasn't. I was extremely logical about what I was going to do.

At the time, I wasn't speaking to any of my family. My siblings wanted to be around but I couldn't deal with a dysfunctional family while I was fighting for my life. I was mentally challenging myself to prepare for this.

When they told me I had metastatic ovarian cancer, they also said I had a 40 percent chance of having kids because I still had a portion of my ovaries. I responded, "Wow, I really want to live." I've had issues with depression and I've been suicidal in the past. All of a sudden, I found I didn't want to die. I would notice the sky and how it looked so blue. There was always this passion and fire inside me. I pulled this strength out of nowhere to get through it and used it to be positive.

In the beginning, the nurses and oncologists were upset with me because I was asking for copies of everything and bringing printouts of articles from the Internet. Later they told me, "You are a model patient. You were so logical with decision-making and you always showed up for chemo." I said, "Of course I'm going to be here; I want to live!" But I found there were people who called in to chemo, like calling in to work, and said, "I'm not going to show up today." As much as I wanted not to go into chemo, I forced myself because I knew how aggressive my cancer was.

I went to chemo nearly every day for about six or seven months. I had no breaks except for the weekends. I was always positive; I listened to music, talked with other patients, and got to know the nurses really well. I was on Facebook a lot and chatted with other cancer survivors.

It connected me with people of all ages and with all types of cancer. That's literally what got me through.

Most of my friends—or people I thought were friends—fell off the face of the earth. It especially scares young people to think of their mortality. I had three acquaintances (Christina was one of them) who were there for me. When I was diagnosed and had surgery, I was immediately put on disability. Christina came over and set up a donation fund, kept track of my medical records, and helped me file for bankruptcy. I'd only known her for six months.

I lost everything, including my apartment and car. But I had friends and my Facebook family to help me through it. Everything fell into place, and I didn't have to do anything but take care of myself. I won't lie, I did have a couple of breakdowns when I was like, "I can't believe this is happening." I think everyone has their down times. But I was always happy. When I woke up, my challenge was to be in the here and now each day and enjoy each moment.

I remember thinking if I can beat this and get to the end of this, I am going to do something that's going to make a difference in people's lives. When I was diagnosed and looking for an ovarian cancer support group on Facebook, I could only find one or two pages. I needed a support group, so I created the Cancer Has Cancer Foundation.

I chose to focus on all cancers; we don't discriminate. One of my friend's brothers was going through colon cancer at the same time I was and at the same hospital. He said, "It doesn't matter; cancer is cancer. It doesn't matter where it is in your body, we need a cure for cancer overall."

"Cure for One, Cure for All" has been the theme for our 5K and everything we do because when you start making progress on one cancer, you eventually start making progress for the rest of them. Through the foundation, we created a Hispanic outreach program. There is a communication barrier for parts of the community, especially older people. Hispanic culture is very fatalistic. You'll hear, "Well if it's my time to go, it's my time to go." It's difficult to explain you need this test; it'll probably save your life.

Once when I was getting chemo, another patient said to me, "You're so calm" in Spanish. I just told her I was just trying to get my mind off of this. I didn't have a port and it was painful. She didn't know why she was there. She didn't even know she had cancer. I looked on cancer organizations' pages and saw only a few things in Spanish, so I saw a need. Cancer is the number one cause of death in the Hispanic community, and no one talks about it.

I held a lot of things in from my childhood. When the cancer happened, I could no longer do that. That is why I've been so open and public about it. I had to talk about it and get it out. That was very therapeutic for me. I started painting, and that was very therapeutic, too. At first the paintings were very dark with a lot of black and gray. Now there are a lot of lighter colors. It's cathartic and soothing. It stops my mind from thinking and reminds me not to worry and be in the moment. I think that's what's really important.

The odds of me living are insane, but I haven't had a recurrence after three years. I have neuropathy, arthritis, and back problems. I'm on a lot of medications. I could be walking in the grocery store, and my leg falls asleep. Before cancer, I used to run six or seven miles and then I would work out. My body has changed. I've joked that I need a walker with tennis balls. But I'm blessed to be here . . . against all odds.

There's been a shift in my life. People who were in my life aren't anymore, but now I have new people, probably the right people. I've also grown closer with my siblings.

I think there are ordinary people who are selected somehow to do extraordinary things and overcome. If I had not gone through such a horrible childhood, I don't think I'd be prepared to handle such a devastating diagnosis and be logical about decisions. Had we not gone to Mexico, I wouldn't have been bilingual. I would not be able to be on Univision giving interviews, or be able to help anyone in the Hispanic community. My past is crazy, but it prepared me for what I was about to embark upon.

I think cancer was a turning point for my life. You can plan all you want, but life has its own plan for you. Everything happens for a reason.

Lessons Learned

- Surround yourself with positive people who will uplift you.
- Live life and be here in the moment now, but let your past be your teacher.
- If you need to cry and vent, you have to do that. Try punching a punching bag, screaming, painting, meditating, Reiki, yoga . . . something that allows you to get emotions out so you can handle it.

To learn more about Heather's foundation, go to the Cancer Has Cancer page (Pinche Cancer en Español) on Facebook, Pinterest, Instagram, and LinkedIn.

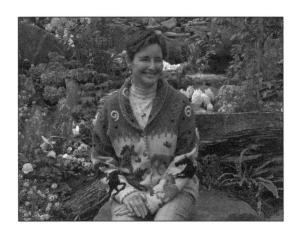

Filling my Cup

Heidi Bright
Cincinnati, OH
Age 53
Diagnosed in July 2009 with stage IV, highly undifferentiated endometrial sarcoma

Cancer was a part of my life at a young age. My mother was diagnosed with breast cancer in 1971 when I was eleven years old. She went in and out of treatment and remission, had multiple surgeries, and died when I had just turned twenty-three.

Her situation was hardly discussed. I don't remember a lot of what happened, yet I remember my dad took over a lot of the cooking. My mother was a very important person to me when I was growing up, and what she said was important. She was not very talkative, so when she told me something, it made an impact on me.

She lived in Berlin during World War II and walked all the way to Heidelberg with her twin sister. They starved one winter. So she was pretty traumatized, and I think that might have influenced her getting cancer.

Although it wasn't the wartime variety, I experienced some stress of my own. I got married in 1989, and we soon started having conflicts. I had two miscarriages early in our marriage and needed fertility treatments to have my first son because I had been unable to get and stay pregnant.

During 2009, my overall stress was worsening. While I was home-schooling my fifth-grader, I also was freelance writing, trying to make enough money to keep my oldest in a private school for gifted children. I would get gigs where I'd end up making $8 to $10 an hour, and I put in a lot of hours. I was always worried about where the next job would come from. I also was trying to eat a paleo (caveman) diet, which involves a lot of prep time.

In March of that year, I noticed I had intermittent bleeding. I was in perimenopause and had a history of endometriosis, so this was not unusual, but I still went to the doctor. She ordered an ultrasound because she noticed there was a mass in my abdomen. The results came back indicating it was a benign fibroid. I understood fibroids tended to disappear after menopause, so I started doing Tai Chi exercises specifically for fibroids and took certain supplements that were supposed to help with it.

But the mass kept growing and growing and growing and, by the end of June, it was getting enormous. We went on vacation in Colorado, and it got so painful that I spent the entire time sitting in the car or hotel, or getting in the hotel bathtub or pool just so I could get some relief from gravity. I called my doctor's office while we were there and told them my symptoms, but was just told the doctor was on vacation. Three weeks later, I finally got a call back. The front office did not understand that my symptoms could be cancerous.

I decided to go to a gynecologist. At this point, I was ready to have a hysterectomy, but because I was a new patient, the gynecologist's office had a three-week waiting period. Every couple of days I called the front office, saying, "Look, these are my symptoms; I really need to get in to see the doctor and get this thing out." Nothing happened.

I wasn't taking pain pills because I wanted to be aware of what was going on. The pain got so bad, I couldn't take it anymore. One night, I woke up my husband to get me to the ER. When we got there, they scheduled me for a hysterectomy and did another ultrasound.

They looked at the results and said it "appeared consistent with sarcoma." I had no idea what sarcoma was. After the doctor explained that it was a type of cancer, I couldn't believe it because I was so healthy otherwise. I had maintained my weight, and I meditated, exercised, and ate right. And I was forty-eight! How could I possibly have cancer?

I didn't know if my fertility treatments had any effect on my getting uterine cancer. During my first pregnancy I had what's called placenta previa, when the embryo plants too low in the uterus and causes bleeding. I have heard that is linked to uterine cancer, but I haven't researched it. At the time, I didn't have time to think about what caused it; we had to take care of it right away.

They switched me over to an oncology surgeon, and I had a nine-hour surgery. They took out my cervix, uterus, tubes, ovaries, and six inches of intestine. They thought it might be stage III because it had gotten outside the uterus. It was sticking to my bladder; it was all over the place. They did a CT scan and found a spot on my lung. They said they weren't sure if it was cancer or histoplasmosis, a kind of fungus that's common in the Ohio Valley.

My sister Roselie, who works for the FDA, had a lot of connections and was able to get me appointments with world specialists in uterine sarcoma at MD Anderson Cancer Center and Memorial Sloan Kettering. Soon we were at MD Anderson, where I got a PET scan that confirmed the spot in my lung was cancer. I had already reached stage IV.

A few weeks later, we went to Sloan Kettering for another opinion. I didn't want to travel for treatment, so my sister found an oncologist in Columbus, Ohio, Dr. Larry Copeland, who was part of the Sarcoma Alliance and had previously worked at MD Anderson. My then-husband and I went to see him after we got back from New York City, and we both agreed this was the perfect person to treat me.

Before we started treatment, I had a baseline scan. It had been six weeks since I had my hysterectomy. In that time, I did what I felt like millions of affirmations, prayed fervently while others prayed for me, meditated an hour a day, and was draconian with my diet. And still, two more nodules showed up in my lungs. I had done all the alternative treatments that I knew of, and still the cancer was growing.

So there was no question, I had to have Western treatment or I was going to be dead. The doctors were quite surprised that my lungs were not full of nodules because that's what they expected with my level of disease. I attribute that to how well I took care of myself, for the most part, before I even got sick.

I did not want to know what my prognosis was—I made that clear to everybody, and nobody told me. I did not want any self-fulfilling prophecies. I also knew that I was not going to be an average patient because I was captain of my fate, not the doctor. My sister later told me I had been given a matter of months to live because of the type and level of cancer I had.

I was open with my sons, then eleven and fourteen, about the cancer because it wasn't done for me when my mother was diagnosed and treated. I understood gaps of information could be filled with imaginary falsehoods, and I didn't want that. I wanted them to know exactly what was going on. They didn't necessarily want to hear it, and they may not remember, but they were told.

I had sixteen treatments of Taxotere and Gemzar. I thought I was doing great and everything was going to disappear, so I skipped my next scheduled scan. But I had a scan in April of 2010 and the cancer was still there. Two of the three nodules had died, but one was actually bigger than it had been in September. Dr. Copeland started me on doxorubicin and cisplatin. I had four treatments and went back for scans four months later. He was very surprised I showed shrinkage already, because with this chemo, it takes that long to just to get started.

I was elated, but after four more months of the combination, a new lung nodule was growing. At that point, the only chemo left was one that required hospital stays. We decided to have the spot surgically removed and send a sample to a lab to do a chemo sensitivity assay, which would determine the best drug for me. We decided to use ifosfamide and Taxol.

I told Dr. Copeland, if I'm going to do hospital-based chemo, I would rather do it in Cincinnati. He recommended oncologist James Pavelka, MD, and I started the regimen. I was in the hospital three days for each treatment, because you run the risk of coma and kidney damage with this type of chemo and they needed to monitor me closely.

I had a scan in May, and it was clean. On July 23, my scan showed a half-inch tumor in the left hilum, next to my heart, sitting right on my pulmonary vein. The oncologist told me he wasn't sure if any surgeon could completely get it out. I called Dr. Patrick Ross, the surgeon in Columbus who performed my first lung surgery, and he seemed pretty confident he could get it.

Within a couple of days, I left my husband because our marriage was stressful. I felt like that was the last resort. I had done everything that I felt was humanly possible to get a cure, and nothing had succeeded. I believed removing this stressful part of my life would possibly give me a fighting chance.

On August 31, 2011, I had the lung surgery. I was supposed to stay in the hospital three to five days, but I was out within two days. It was the same for my first surgery. I credit that to prayer, my lifestyle, and a six-CD set called the "Surgical Support Series" by the Monroe Institute.

You listen to a CD before surgery, during surgery, while in recovery, and when you're in the hospital room. Everybody I've talked to who's used it got out of the hospital a day early.

I couldn't have done the surgery without the support of my friends. They gave me rides to and from surgery, came to the apartment to dress my wounds, took me to the pharmacy, did dishes, and made sure I had food. My sons were teenagers. They weren't running to Mom; they were trying to run off. They are driven at that age to grow up and leave, and yet Mom is sick and needs stuff and wants them to be there. That's hard to deal with when you're a teenager. Rather than rely on them, I tried to rely more on my support system because I had a lot of physical—along with emotional—needs. I tried to spread them out so nobody had to do more than one or two things because I didn't want anybody to get burned out.

Six weeks later when I went for my post-op checkup, a nurse practitioner said the half-inch tumor had grown to two and one half inches during the five weeks between the scan and the surgery. She then told me, "I've been in the cancer surgical department for thirty years, and I see this all the time. You need to either get back on chemo, or get ready for hospice."

There was no more chemo known to be effective against uterine sarcoma. That meant hospice for me. Because of the cancer's aggressiveness and how quickly it came back after such harsh chemo, they expected me to die.

I went back to my apartment and lived with despair for a few days. But then I picked myself back up, got back on my complementary therapies, and focused on just experiencing peace. I went for my next scan six weeks later, and all evidence of disease was gone. My scans have been clean ever since.

I think what helped me most through everything was psychotherapy, which I still do today. My therapist taught me how to manage emotions in a healthy way by simply experiencing them in the moment, inside my body, through a process called the Map of Emotions. My spiritual practices were also very important. I studied theology in seminary and have always been interested in spirituality expressed through the various world religions.

I had already written a couple of traditionally published books and people started encouraging me to write a book about my cancer journey. I thought about it for a long time and realized there are lots of Christian devotionals for the cancer journey, but there's no spiritual reading book that I know about for cancer patients who are not specifically Christian. So I wrote a book called *Thriver Soup: A Feast for Living Consciously During the Cancer Journey*. Each of more than two hundred and fifty entries starts with a reading from one of the world's wisdom traditions, and then I talk about an aspect of the cancer experience related to it and how to apply it to the reader's life.

I share a lot of what I've learned from cancer in the book. Before the diagnosis, I was very stressed about not having time to do things. All my time was absorbed in making sure I was getting everything done for my family and work. It was so bad that I remember one night lying awake for three hours and sobbing the next day because I had lost three hours of my life.

After I was diagnosed, I chose not to stress anymore about getting things done. I decided I needed to be doing what's right for me, not what's right for other people. Before, I was focused on other people's needs and not taking care of what I needed to do for me. Somebody described it this way: It's like you have a teacup, and if you fill it until it overflows, you can give people tea from the saucer. You don't have to give to them everything from the teacup. That's what I'm trying to do today. I fill up my cup so I have something to give to others, rather than giving people an empty teacup.

I believe in the oneness of everything, and I believe that I'm connected with everything. I feel deeply connected with the divine. I guess for me the spiritual lesson is to be who I am, and not who other people want me to be. And if I am who I truly am, that's the best expression of the divine in my life that's possible.

Lessons Learned

- Different things work for different people. I had to figure out what could possibly work for me. I continue to do these practices today.
- For my body, I determined the best diet for me, gently detoxed several times, and exercised.
- Emotionally, in addition to psychotherapy, I would do the Emotional Freedom Technique when I had sudden onsets of fear, despair, and rage. This process involves tapping the ends of all the meridians (a path known in Chinese medicine, through which the life-energy flows) while talking about a specific issue. I wrote in my journal every day about my experiences and my feelings. And I tried to do something every day I really enjoyed and to which I looked forward.
- I had to change my attitude about my life. I had to change my behaviors with other people. And I had to make different choices about what activities I would and would not do.

For more information about Heidi and her book, go to www.heidibright.com.

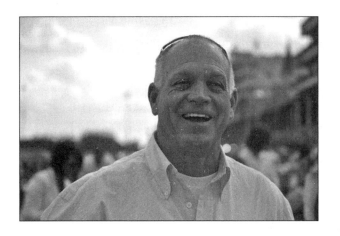

Driven to Thrive

KEN FALHABER
Cincinnati, OH
Age 58
Living with stage IV pancreatic cancer since 2010

It started out in January of 2010. I was fifty-five years old and very active. I worked hard at the car dealership my family owns, played golf, and worked in my yard. The worst thing I'd ever had was getting my appendix taken out and having a meniscus tear. I started feeling sick and thought I had acid reflux or something. I told my brother-in-law, who is my physician, that I just didn't feel right. He ordered test after test, but nothing came up.

In February, they finally did an endoscopy and the doctor told me I had a narrowing of the pancreatic duct, but they didn't see anything else. So I went on and continued to take antacids. The symptoms just got worse, so we did a bunch more tests.

In October, they did another endoscopy. When I woke up from the procedure, the doctor told me I had stage IV pancreatic cancer that had spread to my liver.

I was stunned and amazed. Back in February they found nothing really big, and now stage IV cancer? I asked the doctor, "Okay, how do we fix it? What do we do?" He said that we can't fix it. I said, "You gotta be kidding me! I'm in the car business; we fix everything." He replied, "No, there's no cure; there's nothing we can do except treat you."

I looked over at my wife of thirty-three years, and she had tears running down her cheeks. I knew I was in trouble then.

Growing up, cancer was a word we really never heard or talked about around our house. My mom had early-detected breast cancer years and years ago; no problem. As a matter of fact, this year she's going to be eighty years old. I think my grandmother on my mom's side had passed away of cancer, but she was close to ninety.

Now we had to go home and talk about it with our three adult children. I remember it was a Friday afternoon. I must have looked pretty sick to them because the closing of my bile duct turned my skin yellow. My daughter just hit the ground and couldn't believe it. My second son had lost his first daughter at nine days old almost two years before. So, of course, he was devastated. He was of the mindset, "They took my daughter; they can't take my dad."

That whole weekend was just a blur because all my family members came over to see me. Telling my parents was the hardest thing in the world. Nobody wants to bury their child. I didn't want my parents to have to bury me. My mom was the most worried. I assured them that our family has worked hard all our lives and has never given up on anything. We're not going to start now.

That night, I laid in bed and cried. I looked up to the sky to God and said, "I have no choice over this, but I do have a choice how I react to it. It's not going to control and ruin my life. So if you're gonna call me home, you better get out in front and stop me, because I'm not slowing down."

My brother-in-law told me a few months afterwards, "I didn't think you'd make it through the weekend the way you looked." They took me back in to the hospital on Monday and placed a stent in my bile duct, which brought my coloring back. We met my oncologist on Tuesday and started treatments on Thursday.

Everybody at the dealership just picked up the ball and ran with it because I was devastated. I went into treatment anticipating the worst, praying and hoping for the best, and not knowing what to expect. Everybody was telling me I needed to eat a lot because cancer was going to eat everything off my body. They warned me I'd be fatigued, probably get sick, and lose all my hair—all the negative side effects. I don't hold that against them; they were preparing me for the worst. But I haven't experienced any of the worst.

Within less than a week I started my first treatment with my local oncologist, Dr. Crane. I told him I would like to get additional opinions. He said, "By all means, wherever you want to go, let me know and I'll send all your information to them. I want you to feel comfortable in what you're doing."

We scrambled and went to anyone we could get in front of who would tell me that I had a chance. We went to Indianapolis and talked to people at Indiana/Purdue University. We made two trips to MD Anderson in Houston and traveled to Wisconsin to someone who was considered one of the best pancreatic cancer doctors in the US. We decided to stay with Dr. Crane.

I started out with a drug called Gemzar, which is the protocol drug for pancreatic cancer patients, with a pill called Tarceva. At one point, I switched to what I call "the kitchen sink," about five different medications together which gave me numbness and sensitivity to cold. I couldn't drink anything cold for the first four or five days. Then I had Gemzar and Abraxine, which was a stage 3 trial when I started, but later was approved by the FDA.

In July 2012, I had major surgery to remove my pancreas using the Whipple procedure. It's basically a five-way bypass in which they disconnect your liver, stomach, intestines, gallbladder, and pancreas, take part of them out, and put everything back together again. I lost 10 percent of my stomach, 20 percent of my small intestines, and probably a third of my pancreas. They removed my entire gall bladder.

I was in the hospital for nine days. Two weeks out of surgery, I walked a 2K race for pancreatic cancer at Ohio State.

My body always used to be my temple. If it wasn't low-fat or no-fat, I didn't eat it. I was 5'11" and weighed 170–175 pounds when I was diagnosed. After the surgery, I went down to 140 pounds. I'm still trying to put 10 pounds back on. When you lose part of your pancreas, fats pass through your digestive system pretty quickly. I take enzymes (which the pancreas produces) to keep the fat in me longer so it's absorbed in the body.

But you know what? I had fun getting new clothes, and I've got energy. I feel great. All in all, I've had probably 225 different treatments of chemotherapy and twenty-five radiation treatments, but I eat Mexican food and pizza, drink beer and wine, and am able to do everything I used to do before cancer. But I've been blessed; I've been lucky.

I'm on a clinical trial now because my numbers started escalating a little bit. It's a Phase 1 trial using an agent that's supposed to boost your immune system and stop cancer cells from reproducing. Only 5 percent of all pancreatic cancer patients are eligible for the trial, so I'm fortunate I qualify.

My nurse has told me, "I'm surprised you're still here. You're doing absolutely amazing!" They tell me, for some odd reason, my body is reacting to treatments better than most people and that the cancer is slow-growing.

I've told all my doctors to give newly diagnosed pancreatic cancer patients my phone number and tell them please to call me. I talk to at least one or two newly diagnosed pancreatic cancer patients a month. It's a scary situation, especially when they look up things on the Internet. According to statistics, only 6 percent of patients live for five years. About 74 percent of people die in the first year. They're going to think there's no hope, but I can tell them there is hope. Look at me—I'm a walking vision of hope.

It helped me so much reading success stories on the Pancreatic Action Network's home page. I said, "If they can survive, I can survive, too." Now I'm one of their volunteers and serve as the sponsorship chairperson for the Cincinnati affiliate. Every time someone donates to the organization, a survivor like me thanks them for their donation.

There has not been an increase in the five-year survival rate for the last forty years. It's going to get worse because right now, there's no funding for it. The Pancreatic Action Network was a big part of putting together a recognizant bill that holds the National Cancer Institute liable for developing a strategic plan to improve the five-year survival rate on the four worst cancers.

Part of the problem is that there's no early detection tool, and symptoms don't show up until it's already advanced. I met a young gentleman last year who was fifteen years old and won a corporation's science award for developing a urine test to detect pancreatic cancer that's about 96 percent foolproof. This kid wasn't even of driving age yet; he was a junior in high school. So there is hope for the future.

Most days I don't think about cancer; I just think about today and how I'm going to make somebody else happy and go about my life. But it scares me to death when I think that I might not see my grandchildren grow up. The toughest part about this whole thing is when people talk about the future, because I don't know what the future holds for me, being a stage IV cancer patient. I've lived a great life, though, and I've done all I wanted to do and more.

Because I don't know if there's going to be a tomorrow, if we want to do something, we do it. I still work hard at the dealership, but I play hard now more than I did before cancer. If we want to go somewhere, we go. All I want to do is spend more time with my family and make more memories.

Last year my wife and I celebrated our thirty-fifth anniversary by going to Lake Tahoe, then driving down the coast to Monterey Bay and

Big Sur. We ended up in San Francisco, where we met some family members and walked in the Pancreatic Cancer Walk.

We also bought a villa in Hilton Head, SC, where we go once a month. I told my wife, "I'm not dying, so we might as well enjoy it. And when we both die, our kids can enjoy it for the rest of their lives."

I'm glad my doctors didn't turn the hourglass on me when I was diagnosed, telling me when I was going to die. I didn't ask because I didn't want to know. As far as I'm concerned, they're only doctors. There's only one person who can tell me when it's time to go home, and it isn't a doctor. I wasn't going to give up then and I won't now.

I've always been a determined person, probably to the point of being stubborn. Losing my granddaughter made me a stronger person. Having cancer made me even stronger. I didn't want to die. If I would have given up, I'm sure I would be up in heaven with my granddaughter now. I never pitied myself; I just prayed for time to let other people know that there is hope. That's my mission now.

Lessons Learned

- Attitude makes a difference. Being in the car business, you've got to be positive. That's how my dad has always been, and we've been that way, too. When business is slow, you just tell yourself tomorrow's going to be better. That's how I've handled cancer. Things can be bad, but it can always be worse. Everyone else has their stuff, too.

- Don't give up! There's no one who can tell you how long you have to live beside the Man himself.

- Live life to its fullest. Enjoy everything. If you want to do something, do it. My oncologist told me, "Go live your life and let me handle this." Most people don't give themselves that opportunity unless they are faced with cancer or something else that's life-threatening.

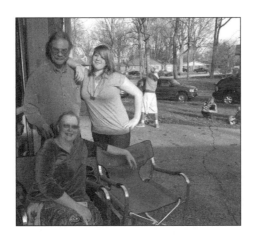

No Expiration Date

Krysti Hughett
Indianapolis, IN
Age 54
Diagnosed in 2004 with stage IV inflammatory breast cancer

I had a wonderful childhood, marred by a few experiences that made me stronger and who I am today. When I was six, I was molested by a friend of the family who went to our church. It went on until my pre-teens when I could get away from him. It was something that, back in the '60s, people didn't talk about. He also molested a classmate and other kids in the neighborhood. He eventually was caught a couple of times, but I wasn't part of that because he threatened to do something to my sister if I told. The more people I talk to about it, the more I realize how it has happened to many people. I think we're more proactive about it now, but it's still hidden a lot.

I didn't repress what happened to me. I think I just made up my mind I wasn't going to let anyone have control over me. When I got to the age when I could change it, I did. If that person came to the house, I would go to my neighbor's house and and hide until he was gone. It made me more proactive and an advocate for me. It made me a stronger person. I wasn't going to let anyone ruin my life. When I was diagnosed with inflammatory breast cancer at age forty-four, I had the same attitude.

I never had a lump, but I noticed both breasts felt larger and had a blush rash on the underside that would come and go. I went to my family doctor, then to a breast center where they did a mammogram and ultrasound, which showed nothing except thicker skin. They did eight core biopsies because I insisted, even though there was no lump to draw from. They didn't believe I had breast cancer. I knew there was something wrong and went to another surgeon.

My mom and I met the new surgeon early in the morning. He told me he never saw anything like my case before. I'm thankful that he sent me to his medical professor, whom we'll call "Dr. Bob," at Indiana University/Purdue University, which is a major medical facility. Dr. Bob called me right after he was out of surgery, and without even an appointment, he said to send me right down to his office.

He examined me and could tell it was inflammatory breast cancer (IBC) right away, but he took two more biopsies. Holding my hand, he said, "This is a serious type of breast cancer, and I'll be with you through thick and thin." He's been my doctor ever since. He calls me his hero, and I call him mine.

I was pretty savvy at the time, but not savvy enough to know there was something called inflammatory breast cancer. We closed the cancer center that day. We went there at 10:30 a.m. and we didn't leave until 6:30 p.m. Dr. Bob introduced me to my oncologist, Kathy, who is a well-known cancer researcher. They worked in a team and included me as part of it from the beginning. They were so good, they told me I should get a second opinion. My mom had called several people for doctor recommendations, and after our appointment she checked her messages. The majority of people recommended Dr. Bob as a surgeon and Kathy as an oncologist. It confirmed we were at the right place.

A couple of days later, my pathology report came back, which showed that along with inflammatory breast cancer, I had invasive ductal, lobular, and comedocarcinoma, a type of invasive ductal carcinoma. So there was a whole spectrum of things going on in both of my breasts.

Originally they thought I was stage III. Two days before my treatment, they did a bunch of scans. There were little spots on my lung. They were too small to do a biopsy.

On Wednesday the next week, I had my port put in. They told me I was going to do chemo first, which was something new at the time. They thought if they did chemo first they could get rid of as many cancer cells as possible. There was no question I'd have chemo and a bilateral mastectomy since it was in both breasts, and inflammatory is so aggressive.

They gave me four dose-dense Taxols, and four dose-dense Adriamycin and Cytoxan (AC) treatments. I used to get worried because people in the chemo room would call AC the "red devil." But I told them, "Hit me as hard as you can; I have children to live for." I was really blessed I didn't get sick and never had to take extra nausea medicine.

I wasn't the kind of person to say, "Just tell me what to do." It frustrates me sometimes when doctors say to not look on the Internet. I get a lot of my information from there. But I can parse out who's selling the fish oil and who's not. I also got a lot of support from the Internet eventually. I learned about inflammatory breast cancer and said, "Oh, I may be in deep doo doo!"

I decided I was going to teach myself as much as I could. Better the beast I knew than I didn't know. I didn't have time to get into a clinical trial. I had to immediately start treatment. Because my oncologist was a researcher, she brought me into the clinical trial world eventually.

I started reading books that would inspire me. The first one was Lance Armstrong's *It's Not About the Bike*. In the beginning, I turned to the Internet and books, not people. I was in the mindset that I can do this myself. I found out Lance was treated at the same hospital. He described in his book where he was put in chemo, and I was so excited. "Wow that's the same chair as mine!" I would say.

My youngest daughter Molly was six and in kindergarten. She was the only kid with the bald mommy. My husband Bill and I decided we were going to be proactive and let her know what was going on. We kept it age-appropriate.

Before I was diagnosed, Molly saw a movie where the mom died of breast cancer. Her first question was, "Mommy, are you going to die?" We said, "We don't know what's going to happen. Mommy is going to fight and hope that nothing like that will happen. Whether something happens or not, you will always be in Mommy's heart, and Mommy's love will always be with you."

I had a hard time looking at my kids and not crying. That's when I made a concerted effort to put one foot in front of another and live in the moment. I learned about living mindfully. My physical therapist had a sign that said, "Breathe, breathe, breathe." That became my mantra.

At the time, there wasn't much known about IBC. That made me mad, so I started on my soapbox. Whenever I was at a teaching hospital, I decided I was going to teach fellows and interns about IBC. I even told the women at the grocery checkout about it. But I thought it was important to know there was an aggressive breast cancer that may not show on a mammogram.

My big thing is to find the blessings, humor, and strength in a situation. It's amazing how many people I had around me; I call them the "angels among us." There were people I didn't even know who reached out and asked what they could do. At first it was hard to answer. A mom from Molly's kindergarten called when I was diagnosed and asked how she could help. I told her I was frustrated that people didn't know about IBC and asked her to forward an email I was going to write about it to her friends. Little did I realize that she was the president of the PTA. So she sent the email out to three hundred and fifty parents.

Interestingly, a few months later, I was in the waiting room to get a scan and started talking to the woman next to me. I joke that I work the waiting room all the time. She asked what I was there for, and I used that opportunity to tell her about IBC. She said, "I got an email about that from a friend!" Eventually I told hundreds of women who were on a couple of email lists and asked them to send the email out to everyone they knew. So they sent it out with attachments about their stories.

One woman named Patty from the west coast had a daughter who was diagnosed with IBC. She was interviewed on a news segment that was shared on the Internet. It led to an entry on Snopes.com to verify that there was such a thing as IBC that was not detectable on a mammogram. I feel proud that it helped people know and that IBC was noted and recognized. It has gone worldwide, and it all started with an email to the president of the PTA.

I had a bilateral mastectomy July of 2005. I wanted the tumor out, my breasts gone. The skin had been affected by IBC so I wanted it off, too. I decided I was going to go flat for the rest of my life. I didn't care about my breasts; they did what they needed to do, and then they tried to kill me.

After I healed, I was to get radiation. Normally radiation is done once a day, but I did some research and learned MD Anderson had an IBC protocol doing it twice a day. I found a female radiation oncologist at a hospital closer to where I live and asked about the protocol. She said, "I'm so glad you asked because I was trained with the MD Anderson protocol. When I first came here, I wanted to do it and nobody would let me."

I told her I would only go there if they would do the MD Anderson protocol, and she said "I'm going to tell my partners I'm going to do this for you." So I started doing radiation at 8 a.m. and 3 p.m. each weekday.

I did 40 regular treatments and eight as a boost that helped bring it to the skin and scar line. The signature characteristic of IBC is that it goes to the scar line often.

I'm someone who, if I don't know something, I will learn about it. I'm going to direct my treatment, not just my doctor. They initially thought I was triple negative, which means you don't have receptors like estrogen or HER2, which was new at the time. While I was doing radiation, I told my oncologist I wanted to do additional testing. She sent the tumor out and we leaned I was HER2 positive. I was able to get the blockbuster drug, Herceptin.

The next summer, I had a CT scan and PET scan and got the results. I was on the way to the American Society of Clinical Oncologists (ASCO) in Chicago, celebrating the news that my PET scan showed that I didn't have any cancer cells in my body. After the conference, however, my oncologist called and said the CT scan showed the spots in my lung were growing.

I was an advocate at ASCO and learned a lot about clinical trials. I decided to choose that path because that's where you find cutting-edge cures. There are different phases of clinical trials. At the time, there were phases 1–4; now there is also phase 0. I do not think clinical trials are a last resort; they should be a first resort and included in treatment options.

Now there are targeted therapies which go directly to cancer cells and sometimes have fewer side effects. I met some people from the National Cancer Institute when I was in advocacy training sponsored by the National Breast Cancer Coalition. That led me to the trial at Vanderbilt in Nashville—a targeted therapy called a PI3 Kinase Inhibitor. PI3 Kinase is a major growth pathway for many cancers. I traveled five hours each way weekly for the trial—close to 100,000 miles. My brother-in-law pointed out that he could have circled the globe three times for all my driving from Indianapolis to Nashville. But it was worth it for me and my family.

I was on the trial for over three years until it stopped working. I just learned a researcher from Johns Hopkins is going to run the breast cancer genome from blood DNA to find out why I have survived so long and did so well on the trial. I'm hoping this will help me and lots of others with the information they find.

I'm now on a trial using Herceptin and Cytoxan with an investigational drug called MM-302, a capsule which contains Adriamycin and antibodies that directly target the HER2 receptor, so it's not attacking healthy cells and causing major side effects. This is my ninth clinical cancer trial. I say I'll always have the next clinical trial in my pocket. I keep my own little database of what's going on both in scientific research from the laboratory bench and on the clinical side, so I can keep an eye on what's looking good.

I feel like the immune system is really important. I figure I'll use all my options. I do all kinds of complementary therapies, such as meditation and yoga. I have used supplements but I'm really careful about it and research them on web pages, like "About Herbs" from Memorial Sloan Kettering's website.

Once I was diagnosed with stage IV, I reached out more for support. It's probably harder for my family than it is for me at times. I'm the one who's in the fight and do what I need to do. Sometimes they're scared, and that doesn't help them deal with it. Through the Cancer Support Community (CSC), I was able to get support for me and my family.

Everyone deals with cancer differently. My youngest was my cheerleader and supporter. My oldest daughter was in freshman year of college. She went into denial and didn't want to know or hear about it. Later, we talked about it and she told me she was scared. My middle daughter, my stepdaughter, was in California living with her mom at the time. She called me once or twice a day.

My husband wanted to fix it. It's frustrating for our spouses who realize they can't fix it, especially when you're metastatic. I found this book early on at the CSC called *Breast Cancer Husband*. It helped me realize there are different ways to cope.

I also found out about a camp called Camp Kesem for Molly. It has been a godsend; this will be her tenth year going. It's free for kids with a parent with cancer whether they're in treatment, out of treatment, or passed away from cancer.

I have learned so much from advocacy work. It helped me to meet researchers, go to scientific conferences, and understand my oncologist. My oncologist has come to these conferences, and when she introduces me to other oncologists she jokes, "Watch out, she knows more about breast cancer than I do."

Stage IV breast cancer isn't curable, but I think I've made it more of a chronic disease. I truly think there will be not one but many cures for stage IV breast cancer. We know there are a thousand genes involved in breast cancer alone. And it's different for everyone; it might not just be a mutation.

I think keeping really positive has been an important thing for me along this journey. Sadly, I know a lot of positive breast cancer warriors who have not survived. But for me, it has helped me. I buy two-year calendars because I plan on being here. When I was first diagnosed with stage IV, I probably had a very short time to live. My doctors never gave me a time limit. I think that was important. They said to me that they'd let me know if I was closer to needing to make any arrangements.

Through the years, I've had eleven brain tumors. I had one little tumor we got with gamma knife surgery a year ago. There are some people who think, *If I have a brain tumor, it's all over.* Sometimes I go there, but part of living with this disease is not letting that thought take over.

When I was diagnosed with the first brain tumor, I had to carefully tell myself, "This is not the end." For almost four years, brain tumors popped up and we zapped them with radiation. It's one of the easiest things I've ever done, but it looks kind of scary when they screw a metal halo to your head and put you in a machine. I have to calm myself with breathing and repeat, "Never give up." I've done four gamma knife procedures overall.

At one point, I was NED (No Evidence of Disease). I call it No Expiration Date. When my husband got me a handicapped sticker—which I needed because I had a brain tumor at the time—it said "No expiration." That's what I focus on whenever I'm in my car. I want to stamp that on my forehead. I'm not accepting that cancer will kill me, although I know it's a possibility.

One time, I was giving a speech and I realized I had lived through all my milestones on my list. I thought, *I need to have more and make them further out.* I fully expect to see a grandchild at one point. I joke that I'm going to get an old lady's breast cancer that's going to get slower and slower, and I'm going to get faster and faster. I think that's part of living with hope.

Life Lessons

- Live with hope. I found a quote that you can live a certain time without food, and certain time without water, but you can't live two seconds without hope.

- Seek help and information. There are many sources for information: Annie Appleseed Project (complementary treatments), IBC Research Foundation, and findings from the annual San Antonio Breast Cancer Symposium in December.

- Don't rule out clinical trials. I use *www.clinicaltrials.gov* and *www.bctrials.org*—databases that allow you to enter your information, so they can send you information about trials for which you qualify. Center Watch is another resource.

- Don't let cost be a factor. I didn't know to ask in the beginning, but I learned to ask and find out. I don't just say, "Hey, the logistics won't work for me." I research the options. The Patient Advocate Foundation is a great resource to find out about financial help. There are a lot of organizations that assist with travel costs and co-pays.

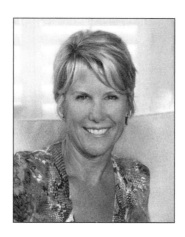

Invent Your Own Miracle

Laurie Beck
Santa Rosa Beach, FL
Age 50
**Diagnosed in 2006 with incurable Non-Hodgkin's lymphoma
and marginal cell leukemia**

Starting at twelve and up to my early forties, I had chronic stress. I didn't realize how chronic it was until I got sick. The irony behind that is, my mom, Loretta LaRoche, has written ten books and speaks all over the world . . . on the topic of stress. She's probably one of the best stress gurus in the country.

I started emotionally eating at age twelve when my parents divorced. On the outside, everything looked so idyllic. I spent my summers in the Hamptons with my grandparents and went to a highly regarded boarding school. But the truth was that my mother was working three jobs to make ends meet and my brothers and I found ways to get in trouble. I suffered from anxiety and always felt so ashamed and not worthy.

My mother and grandparents were amazing Italian cooks, and food was my way of making me feel good. Granny was always infusing us with homemade pasta, and she made the most incredible pizza you could ever eat. My eating went out of control and I became bulimic. When I met my first husband at age nineteen, I lost all the weight in six months and never gained it back. I learned if I moved my body, I could help alleviate stress and lose weight in the process. If I did some form of exercise for one hour, it was almost like taking a pill for me.

When my sons were two and four, my husband was taken away to federal camp for five years. I really never knew what took place but he was involved in a scam, similar to what happened in the movie *Catch Me if You Can*. I was living what I thought was my dream life, and it was taken away.

We divorced and I soon remarried to my wonderful husband Bob. My life became stable again until my ex got out of prison. He started following me, and then he ended up going back again. Every time this happened, he was hurting the children.

All of the shame and sadness weighed on me. When my son turned fourteen, he started getting in trouble, so we decided to move from Atlanta to Florida to try to prevent him from going down a bad path. Several years prior to this we took in my stepson, then had my eighty-nine-year-old granny live with us. She had Parkinson's disease and, later, dementia, and couldn't live by herself anymore. Some family drama ensued, which led to Granny going to a nursing home and me being estranged from my mother. I think there was chronic, constant stress that never allowed me to just be Laurie.

Luckily I found Pilates. I loved how it made me feel and taught me how to breathe. I became certified, and opened up a studio at the beach. A year later, I noticed a rash under my right arm. I always avoided doctors and dismissed the rash as skin irritation from exercise. After three months of seeking advice, self-diagnosing, and making excuses, I finally broke down and went to a dermatologist. Two doctors and several skin creams later, the rash had not subsided.

After much urging, I felt around and discovered two lumps, one deep in each armpit, and later three additional lumps on the back of my neck. My left rib cage felt sore, but I continued to ignore the warning signs. Eventually, I couldn't get through the day without a nap or gasping for breath when taking the stairs. Six months passed by the time Bob finally persuaded me to see my doctor.

After an extensive blood panel and a bone marrow biopsy, I learned I had a rare form of Non-Hodgkin's lymphoma and marginal cell leukemia, which was incurable. My spleen was enlarged, about 65 percent of my lymphatic system was compromised, and I had tumors in multiple places. They told me I needed to immediately start an aggressive chemotherapy regimen. I went for another opinion and I heard the same diagnosis and recommendation.

I decided to go to Dana Farber in Boston to see one more doctor. Unlike the other two doctors, he recommended watchful waiting. He said, "If we don't see a change in this, we will need to take out your spleen and put you on chemotherapy." I gathered as much information as I could to understand what the chemo was going to do instead of waiting three months and trying other things. I went with my gut and I decided to follow his advice.

I could hear buzz around me. A lot of people were questioning my decision. My husband begged me to consider chemo because he wanted it knocked out of my body. One of my good friends was the head oncology nurse at the first hospital where I received my diagnosis. She read my doctor's findings and was horrified that I chose to wait instead of going with what the oncologist recommended.

I felt confused and scared and needed an ally. My mom became very well-known and was traveling two to three times a week for speaking engagements. I knew she was exhausted, and we hadn't spoken to each other for three years. It took me a very long time, but I'm so grateful I dialed her number. After that conversation, she became my biggest advocate. I feel strongly she helped saved my life.

The day before my appointment at Dana Farber, she booked me for appointment with her Reiki master. I had to fly from Florida to Boston, where she lived, and I thought, *What the heck is a Reiki master?* But I repeated the mantra, "What do I have to lose?"

She dropped me off at this appointment and I got on the table and I closed my eyes. I didn't take my clothes off and the woman was not even touching me. I thought, *This is really weird*, and then she lit sage and swept it around me. When the session ended, I opened my eyes, and, I felt so different.

She said, "My hands were not going to leave the left side of your body and your lung area." She didn't know my spleen was very compromised and I had tumors in my lungs. That fascinated me.

As we were leaving to get on the plane after we did all our tests at Dana Farber, Mom looked at me and said, "Okay, go get acupuncture." I looked back at her and said, "Mom, I have cancer." She replied, "I know, I want you to go get acupuncture. It will help with blockage and stress in your body."

I will never forget on May 18, 2006, I walked into my first acupuncture appointment. It was a life-changing experience. From there, I began doing traditional Chinese medicine. For three years, I drank a formula designed for me. It looked like dirt and bark and tasted nasty, but I drank it and called it my healing potion.

I dramatically cut back on my work at the Pilates studio and focused 100 percent on healing my body, mind, and spirit. At first, I had no clue what it was doing, but each time I went to the doctor for scans and blood work, my results were better. This confirmed to me that I was doing the right thing and stayed the course. I never went on chemo.

Despite all of the things I was doing, pessimism still crept in. I realized I needed to heal my spirit before I healed my body. One of my former clients referred me to an energy healer who helped me let go of the resentment from my past that was still affecting my relationships.

I learned how to "Shift my stinkin' thinkin'," as my mom would say. There would be days that I would terrorize myself, wondering if I was going to live or die. My mom taught me to go to the worst place and shift it to a happy place and be in the moment. Once I learned this, I could feel my body relax and feel things shifting.

One time when she was going with me to get a CT scan, she noticed how my body tensed in the elevator. I was claustrophobic, which was made even worse when we came down to the hospital basement. There were no windows, and I was looking for a way out. When we got to the CT scan, I read signs on the wall. In my mind, I interpreted them as saying, "Once you go in that room, you're never going to come out of it again."

My mom looks at me, and she says, "What is wrong with you?" And I say, "These signs, I'm reading them, and they're scaring the daylights out of me!" She replies, "Well, stop reading them!" It was brilliant and that re-shifted my thinking so I could get over my claustrophobia and do my CT scan.

In May 2009, I went in for my blood work and everything was clean. I had no evidence of cancer. I continue to get checked. That's something I have to do for the rest of my life. I don't ever get the cancer card where it goes away. But the cancer is still "in the closet."

I still do acupuncture and Reiki and Pilates, but the most powerful thing I've done is to keep negative influences out of my life. I try to be really positive and careful about who I surround myself with so I don't overextend myself and create things that aren't good for me.

Sometimes you have to invent your own miracle. Every scenario is different. Not everyone can do what I did. You can do a complementary approach that combines traditional and alternative therapies. Of course you have to make sure whatever you do is okay with your doctor, but you need to become a part of your doctor's team.

I firmly believe you can't just cut the cancer out of you, do some chemo or radiation, and think you're done. Cancer can also take over your mind, spirit, and your body, so you have to heal all three to get rid of it. You have to live, eat, and breathe positive intention. You have to find a way to forgive so that healing can begin, and search every day to find serenity. And you need to make sure that you are throwing every healing modality—Western, Eastern, and otherwise—at that disease in your body.

Lessons Learned

- You need to surround yourself with as much positivity and love as possible. You can't eliminate all stress, but figure out ways to cope better with whatever stresses are going on in your life.
- Find a way to bring spirituality into your life. The power of prayer is huge. It can be as simple as waking up in the morning and being thankful or saying, "Thank you for this moment."
- Get a second opinion, and not just a second opinion anywhere. There are hospitals that specialize in very specific cancers. When I went to the first hospital, I asked, "How many cases have you worked with or seen like mine?" The doctor replied, "In the fifteen years, I've only seen three to five cases." When I went to Dana Farber and I asked that same question, the doctor said, "We are seeing two to three hundred cases a year."

Laurie Beck is a mom, certified Pilates instructor, wellness expert, Reiki practitioner, coach, jewelry designer, horse trainer, and author of I Am Living to Tell. *For more information, go to* www.lauriebeck.com.

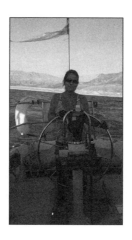

Adventures at Camp Chemo

Lynda DeWitt
Los Angeles, CA
Age 52
Diagnosed in 2002 with stage IV, HER-2, and estrogen/
progesterone-positive breast cancer

My dad was quite the character. He and his brother decided in the late 1960s that they should build a boat and go sailing around the world. But pretty much anytime we went anywhere, parts of the boat broke because they weren't boat builders. I was a kid and saw it as an adventure. I remember approaching an island in the middle of the ocean and being told there was something wrong and we might be going in the water. "You just hang tight and wait for a helicopter to come rescue you," my dad told me. I thought, "Yay! I'm going swimming!"

When I got married in 1990, it was to a man who shared my love of traveling and sailing. And once again, I was living on a boat. We had lots of fun for several years, but eventually I found myself in some choppy waters.

In the spring of 2002, I was forty and I was about to start a new job opening a new retail store and knew it was going to be busy all through the summer. So I decided I was going to get all my checkups, including my mammogram that wasn't due until six months, so I wouldn't have to take time off.

I had my mammogram in April, and I got a letter telling me they found something suspicious. This had happened plenty of times because I have fibrous breasts and had fibroid tumors. I had one removed back in the late '80s, but it was benign. So, I was kind of used to those types of letters after a mammogram.

On May 3, I went in for another mammogram and had a needle biopsy right there. That had never happened before. I knew by the expression on the girl's face when she did the needle aspiration that something wasn't right.

I got a call from the surgeon on May 7, saying that I had breast cancer and that I needed to see an oncologist right away. I started chemo on the 13th, that following Monday; they didn't wait at all. They wanted to do chemo first to shrink the tumor. In some cases, if you removed the tumor first and then did chemo, you couldn't tell if it was working or not because the tumor was gone.

The normal protocol for my type of cancer was Adriamycin, Taxotere, and Cytoxan. But my oncologist, Dr. John Link, was doing groundbreaking research and changing protocols for women like me— premenopausal with extremely aggressive HER2-positive cancer. He discovered, along with other colleagues around the world, it really worked a lot better in cases like mine if you separated the three drugs, doubled the dose, and gave it in half the time. So that's what they did.

I've never been one to think of new situations as scary or depressing. I just have this innate ability to see the positive in everything, and I've been this way my whole life. I remember the first day going to treatment thinking, *Yay, Camp Chemo!* To me it was just a new experience.

I had great trust in my doctors and knew I was in a good place. And honestly, because I was so ignorant to what cancer really was, I didn't have the fear. I didn't realize at the time how hard it was going to be. I never stayed up late nights thinking, *Oh, I'm going to die from this.* That wasn't until much later.

The day I was diagnosed, I went to get my hair cut and had them give me a purple Mohawk. I never cut my hair, so it was very long—down to my waist. I always wanted a purple Mohawk, but I didn't want the maintenance of it. But this was my one opportunity because I knew it was going to be gone in a couple weeks.

It set the tone for my adventure because I'd learned some things from that Mohawk. I had to walk to the end of the dock every day to get to my boat. I knew a lot of my neighbors, but we weren't really friends. It's a hard thing to walk up to your neighbors and say, "Hey, you know, I got cancer." How do you start that conversation with acquaintances?

The Mohawk did it. People saw me on the docks and went, "Whoa, what the hell did you do?" It gave me the opportunity to tell people about the cancer, while letting them see that I still had my sense of humor. I teared up a little when I was saying it because at the time everything was so raw, but it was such an easy way for them to accept it. It was an opening for the conversation.

Also on the day I was diagnosed, I found a pamphlet for Breast Friends, a mentoring program that matches you with another survivor who has a similar diagnosis and treatment. I've never been one to suffer in silence, so I called them immediately and said, "Give me a mentor!" I was able to call her any time day or night with questions, and it really made a difference.

In September, after eighteen weeks of the strongest chemo I could receive, they removed the tumor. My surgeon told me the tumor had spider-like legs that went out and wrapped around nerve endings, blood vessels, and anything else in its path, so it was really hard to remove all of it. Scans showed cancer in distant lymph nodes and some suspicious spots in my liver, and I learned I had stage IV cancer. I didn't know stage door from stage IV; I didn't know anything about it.

After my surgery, they also sent off pathology to a lab for chemo-sensitivity testing to determine which chemotherapy agents the cancer responded to. The study showed my cancer was most sensitive to Navelbene and Taxol, so I did four more months of the dose-dense combination.

In November, I started accidentally falling into the boat because I couldn't feel my feet anymore from the neuropathy. A sailboat is a tricky place; it's kind of like living under your dining room table. It's great when you're out at the islands and you're traveling, but when you're sick from chemo . . . the smells and the mold made me miserable. I didn't have running water or refrigeration, and I had to shower in the marina public shower, and that was never good. I had to grocery shop and buy ice every day. And my husband was a truck driver so he was out of town a lot.

Everyone was saying, "You have to move off the boat if you're going to survive the winter!" But my husband wasn't going to have any part of that. He loved living on the boat, and that was his life. The third time I fell into the boat, I was carrying groceries and slid all the way down and ended up flat on my back on the floor. My leg was twisted back and I was surrounded by broken glass. I remember a tiny voice in my head said, "You're going to survive this cancer, but you won't survive a broken neck."

My parents live a hundred miles away, so I couldn't move in with them and continue treatment with my doctor. I had friends willing to take me in, but it wasn't going to be easy for any of them; I didn't want to be a burden. I went to a social worker and called the American Cancer Society and Komen, but no one could help me find a place to live.

I told my nurse practitioner about the situation, and she gave me a pamphlet for Breast Cancer Angels. I called their number, and a lady named Faye Dietiker answered. She was the director and founder. I told her my story and was probably a blubbering idiot. I was scared I was dying, and even more scared I was going to lose my husband after I moved off the boat. After about twenty minutes of my sad story, she said "Honey, you find a room, and we'll pay your rent." For eighteen months, they paid my rent. They also gave me two hundred dollars in grocery gift certificates. I couldn't believe it. I don't think I could have survived without their support.

A friend of mine knew a man named Ron who had a big beautiful house and gave me two rooms and a bathroom that were closed off from the rest of the house. So on December 22, 2002, before I was even done with treatment, I moved off the boat and into this beautiful little oasis. The backyard was like the Garden of Eden. It had a fountain, and I would sit outside and watch the birds.

I had a bathroom and a bathtub, where I could soak when I was sore from chemo. I had a real kitchen and could actually keep things in the freezer. I had a laundry machine right there; I didn't have to go to the laundromat. It was heaven to me.

I started going to Breast Cancer Angels monthly support meetings. I learned a lot . . . that not all doctors treat you the same and not all cancers are the same. And I learned how fortunate I was to have a doctor who treated me aggressively because I started losing friends who didn't even have cancer as aggressive as mine.

After I completed radiation, just a couple of weeks before my one-year anniversary, my doctor told me, "Go live your life." But about a month later, I was in the hospital with a staph infection. That's what almost did me in because I had no immune system to fight it.

On Memorial Day weekend, I noticed my left breast was bright red and rock-hard. I went to Urgent Care, and they said I had an infection and gave me a shot of something. It didn't work; my head was pounding and everything hurt. I went to my oncologist who gave me another shot, but it still didn't work. On May 30, they admitted me to the hospital, and gave me a hard-core antibiotic.

I started feeling better, so they sent me home with a regimen of antibiotics. Four weeks later, my surgeon noticed a rash on my stomach during a follow-up appointment. She told me, "Stop the antibiotics now." A few days later, I had rashes over my entire body and was having problems breathing. They took me right to the hospital, where they lanced my breast and found a staph infection had gotten into an empty cavity where the tumor had been, and colonized.

At that point, my immune system just threw in the towel. The antibiotic broke down my capillaries so my fingertips and toes started bleeding out. I was just being poisoned, and my body had no reserves to fight it.

I was in the hospital from Monday the 7th of July through Sunday the 20th. When I got home from that, I might as well have been a vegetable; I was so weak and tired. And that's when everything started going sideways. I woke up one night with an eye occlusion that looked like the continent of Africa. My ophthalmologist told me cancer had returned in the eye, but my oncologist confirmed it was caused by the antibiotic pooling behind it.

They finally got rid of the staph infection, but I start having serious allergy issues. Every day I woke up and couldn't stop sneezing. I went to see an allergist, who tested me for sixty-six things, and I was allergic to all but two of them. So they started me on steroids and other medications.

One Saturday, I was putting out balloons for an event. It was my coworker's birthday so I sucked a little helium out of a balloon and sang "Happy Birthday." A minute later, my lungs shut down, and they called the ambulance because I couldn't breathe. At first they thought my lungs collapsed, but they found out I was now allergic to latex.

Every time something like that happened, a doctor told me my cancer was back. They would just look at my chart and see I had cancer, so they would assume it was cancer-related. It was a rollercoaster year, going through all that weirdness. I somehow got through it, but my marriage didn't fare as well. We parted, fairly amicably, in 2004.

I decided to go to college so I could find a job and support myself. Even though we were separated, my husband agreed to stay married so

I could stay on his insurance. I believed if I didn't have his insurance, I wouldn't be here today. He had really good insurance; it paid for everything. But it was heartbreaking, because I knew ladies who didn't have insurance or had crappy insurance.

My doctor told me about a vaccine program that was going on in Seattle. It was a government program for HER2-positive tumors, and I was a perfect candidate. In July 2005, I made my first trip to Seattle and got the vaccine over the next year and a half. I've been in remission ever since.

I was the tenth of sixty-six women to get the vaccine. I felt like a pioneer and empowered, knowing I might help prevent breast cancer for my daughter and other young women. I believe cancer vaccines are the wave of the future. If your immune system is at its optimum, I think you can fight cancer. This vaccine teaches your immune system to fight off cancer. Here I am eleven-plus years later. I think there are a lot of contributing factors to my success, but the vaccine has done the most to keep me alive this long and to keep my cancer so non-aggressive.

The vaccine is still in an ongoing study. It takes many years to gather all the information. The beauty of the vaccine is that if, and probably when, my cancer does come back, I can go get a booster vaccine. For peace of mind, you need a couple of cards up your sleeve.

My greatest gift was having the right doctors. When I mentor new patients now, I tell them to do the research, get a second opinion, and find the best doctor. When my daughter was in school and had a teacher she liked, she did so much better in the class. When you have a doctor you like and trust, I believe you do so much better in the treatment.

I'm still in treatment. I do Herceptin every three weeks and I take a pill every day called Femara. My oncologist watches me like a hawk. Every three months, I get scanned and tested. Last month, I had my mammogram and a lymph node on the right side showed up suspicious. I went in for another biopsy and I learned the results were benign.

Luckily, I don't play the "what if" game negatively. If I play that game, it's always a positive outcome. I have a biopsy. Am I losing sleep over it? Nope. It is what it is, and I could fall apart and lose it, but it's not going to make any difference.

The first time I had chemo, I visualized bulldozers taking buckets of Adriamycin to the cancer site, and then dumping them on top of the cancer to make me cancer-free. They were like my little army inside me. I still visualize treatment doing what it's supposed to do. I'm not one to sit in a chair and go, "This isn't working," because to me that's counter-productive. If you're going to get positive results, you've got to put in positive input.

I think sailing has taught me to be like this. It's an interesting sport with long periods of sheer nothingness, boredom almost, followed by extremely short bursts of panic-stricken moments. You can be sailing for days and days and nothing's happening. Then something will break or something happens—usually in the middle of the night when you're sleeping. So I learned early on when that kind of stuff happens to mellow it out. I think sailing taught me to focus and not get weird in a panic situation.

I am fortunate to have someone in my life who is there for me. In 2005, I met Stan. We were both going through a divorce, and I really didn't have any want or need for a romantic relationship. But we talked a lot and we both were going through hard times. For a year, we were just really good friends and then it progressed from there. In 2010, we got married.

I'm a grandma now. My grandson, Grayson, is six, and my grand-daughter, Andie, is three. They call me "Grambo" because I'm part Grandma, part Rambo. When they come spend the night, we do what they want to do. They want to go to the park, we go to the park. They want to crack eggs, we bake something. I have the time to make them the center of attention when they're with me.

We went to the LA County Fair on Saturday. Grayson won a fish and a ton of stuffed animals. We had so much fun. I don't want cancer to ever keep me from doing the things I want to do. I really don't want anything to keep me from doing the things I want to do. My life is an adventure waiting to unfold, and as long as I'm here, I'm going to live it to the fullest.

Lessons Learned

- Doctors are dealing with thousands of patients. And every single cancer is unique to that person. You have to be proactive and be your best advocate. You have to ask questions, and if you don't get the answer you want or you can't understand, ask again. If you still aren't getting what you want, go someplace else.
- Don't ever give up hope. Sometimes I think doctors want to give you the worst case scenario so you're not disappointed when it doesn't work out. Or they're just so glazed over from what they have to deal with every day. But they don't know . . . and I'm living proof of that. Luckily I never had any doctor say, "Well, you're going to die; you need to get your affairs in order." My doctor said to me from the very beginning, "This is going to be hard, but we're going to fight this, and I'm going to see you through this."
- Reach out for help. There are organizations dedicated to helping cancer survivors, and friends and family can help, too..But you have to ask and look for resources.

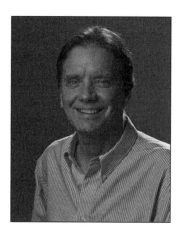

Lifelines to Cancer Survival

Mark Roby
Detroit, MI
Age 59
Diagnosed in 2002 with stage IV epithelioid hemangioendothelioma (a rare type of liver cancer)

I began an inner healing journey while working as a physician's assistant at a large medical center north of Detroit. My mom, older sister, and I had experienced headaches most of our lives. I was a workaholic and put a lot of stress on myself. I started getting headaches, and also started developing serious heart problems. Holistic healing was growing in popularity throughout the United States and I decided I wanted to do healing work on myself.

I met with Dr. Jerry Jampolsky, the founder of Attitudinal Healing, a movement out of California that helps people going through health and life challenges. He asked me to start a Center for Attitudinal Healing here in Michigan, and it's still going. A lot of people with cancer, depression, and other illnesses come through our groups and seminars to learn meditation and other inner healing philosophies.

As time went on, working on me took a back seat to helping others. In the fall of 2002, I was consulting with the center while putting in countless hours at the hospital. I got engaged to a woman who lived out of town in Traverse City and spent a lot of time traveling back and forth to see her. I was burnt out and exhausted.

My whole life, I've been a runner, so I ran every night after work. I didn't take any nights off, even when I traveled. I also lifted weights. I started getting a pain in my side, but I thought, "I'm in my late forties; I'm just burnt out and pulled a muscle."

I had forgotten it at the time, but I had a recurring dream with a voice telling me that I was in danger and should go to see the doctor. Even though I practically lived in hospitals, I didn't like going to see the doctor or taking medicine. I had just completed my Doctor of Naturopathy degree and wasn't in that mindset.

Everything came to a head in December. I was exhausted, losing weight, and having fevers. I was going to go up north to Traverse City after working ten days straight. It was snowing, and I came home to take a three-mile run. Toward the end, I felt this pain in my right side. And then when I got in my condo, I just collapsed on the floor and could hardly get up. The pain was so bad I couldn't breathe, and my belly and chest hurt. So I lay on the floor and called my fiancée. She yelled at me to get to the hospital.

It was hard to do, but I got myself in the car and went to the ER where I worked. It was a smaller institution and they weren't sure what was going on, so they sent me to a huge medical facility on the outskirts of Detroit. They did scans and kept me overnight. I called my dad and he was there when I got the news. In the morning, the doctor just came in and said, "You have cancer all over your liver and your lungs."

My dad held me and we both cried. I was pretty delirious because I was so sick, which made matters worse. The doctor explained they thought the cancer originated somewhere else in my body and that they were going to keep me for a while to do tests. He said, "It doesn't look good."

They kept me for five or six days and did all kinds of tests, but they couldn't find the etiology. On the fifth day, they did some biopsies. All they gave me was a little local anesthesia. They couldn't get into my liver from my abdomen because it hurt so much, so then they went in through my chest. I was in such agonizing pain; I had to bite on a tongue depressor they gave me and squeeze a nurse's hand.

On New Year's Day in 2003, the oncologist came in and said, "Well, we finally have an answer. You have a very rare type of sarcoma that started in your liver called epithelioid hemangioendothelioma. There are only two short paragraphs in the oncology book about it. We think it's in your bones and your lungs. I'd probably give you about six months to live. I'm sorry."

He recommended I go see the head oncologist at University of Michigan then come back with the treatment plan, and that was it.

One of my friends referred me to some contacts around the country. Before I left the hospital, I called a liver surgeon at Sloan Kettering. We talked for a while, and I told him everything about my case. He said to me, "Mark, I'm sorry to tell you, there's no hope. It sounds so advanced you can't be operated on."

I hung up the phone. Then my fiancée came down and took me out to see *Lord of the Rings*. I laid on her lap because I was exhausted. I didn't really see the movie; it was almost like a dream. I was so weak and in horrible pain; I was just trying to make it through each day.

I think the two things that saved me at the time were one, I had an extensive group of friends and colleagues from Attitudinal Healing and in the medical field who were trying to find answers to my medical issues. And two, God helped me. I didn't have any answers then, but within a month or two, God was talking to me in different ways, telling me that He would show me a way through it.

I loved to work, but my job in the ER was so stressful. I talked with my friends for a few weeks, and it was decided as a group that it would be ridiculous for me to try to work. Unfortunately, I had just declined a disability policy a year or two earlier because I never got sick prior to this.

It took me a few weeks, but finally I realized surviving would be job Number One. I had some savings and good insurance, which helped. I was really lucky to have friends and colleagues who did a lot of fund-raisers for me. From the first few months they knew I was in trouble, people from all over the country helped me.

I sought tons of opinions. After talking with an oncologist from Sloan Kettering, my doctor said they would try interferon, but they didn't know if it'd work or not. They were just going to give me interferon palliative therapy to try to stave it off. I went to three other hospitals for opinions. And then I went down to a prominent cancer center in another state. I was supposed to be there for just a week. They kept me for four weeks as an outpatient. They lost my slides and records and took vacations without telling me, and ran through my money like water. After that, they told me the same thing I heard from my local oncologist: I was probably going to die, but interferon might stave it off. They suggested I go on ten million units every other day, which is an ungodly amount.

So when I came back home, my initial oncologist started on the plan. After six weeks, it wasn't working. While I was getting the therapy and was really sick, he'd whisper to me, "Mark, nothing we're doing is going to help, so you might as well just accept it. We could try Avastin, Sutent, and a myriad of new drugs, but nothing is going to work. I don't know why you're going all over the country. Why don't you just enjoy the few months you have left, and take a vacation with your fiancée or something."

I could only take seven or eight weeks of treatment before I landed in the hospital. I was sicker than a dog; I couldn't function. My friends helped me function at home, even bathing me. Some people actually commit suicide when they're on those high doses of interferon because it's just devastating. Even if you're on two or three million units, you can really feel it. But to be on ten million units, that's a pretty high dose.

I was dizzy, felt faint, foggy, exhausted ... you name it! And my medical bills were mounting to astronomical amounts.

Everyone I had encountered in the medical community was convinced I would die, except for one person. I talked with a medical researcher who told me I might live and how to do it. To keep myself alive, he said I had to come up with three contingency plans. I call it the triad of survival. Once Plan A stopped working, I had to go to Plan B. Then if Plan B didn't work, I would go to Plan C. But I had to always find new plans so I would have three at all times. I'm still following his advice eleven years later and recommending it to patients I help. Currently, I'm on my third triad of survival.

Another survival strategy has been my diet. The typical American diet is comprised of a lot of protein, fat, and sugar. After they're metabolized, they have acidic residual, kind of like exhaust, with a lot of free radicals that promote cancer. So going in, I knew that I had to do the opposite of that. I started a strict diet of vegetables, alkaline water, berries, and foods rich in Omega 3 fatty acids like nuts, avocados, and fish.

I did a lot of research on inflammation and angiogenesis, keeping folders with information that I brought to my doctors. Very few of them would listen to me really, or even take it seriously. They just told me to eat anything I want and that I should eat a lot of protein, like meat and ice cream. And they warned me that the herbs and vitamins I was taking were dangerous. I just did the complete opposite of everything they told me!

I learned more and did everything to try to make my body cancer unfriendly. I still do every day. Over the years, I tried a combination of traditional and natural treatments. In 2009, I had a liver transplant. In the summer of 2011, while I was still on the immunosuppressant drugs to keep my body from rejecting the liver, the cancer came back. They put me on chemo, but it kept spreading. I went to Boston to get a genetic profile of my tumor; it came back as positive for mTOR, a major pathway for the growth of many solid tumors. I opted for radiofrequency ablation in December of that year and started on

Rapamycin. It's one of the new targeted anti-cancer drugs that suppress the mTOR pathway. I've been clear of cancer since.

I've leaned heavily on God and Jesus since the onset, and I'm not ashamed to say that I give them the credit first. I think God works through people. That's the purpose of life—helping each other. I think that cancer brings out the best and the worst in situations.

When doctors were giving me no hope year after year, my faith got me through it. I gave my worries to God, who guided me to go after the cancer physically, mentally, and emotionally. I knew I had to go on a full frontal attack.

Ten years ago, when I thought I was dying, I had long conversations from my hospital bed with Jerry Jampolsky. He told me, "Mark, you know, your purpose is to help people." I'm on the earth not to sit around and be an observer, but to take action.

When I was stuck at that cancer center for weeks on end, I started volunteering in the hospital. I pushed patients around and gave them directions and tried to help the parents and their children who had cancer. It took my mind off myself and gave me a purpose. When I was back in Michigan, I worked in the soup kitchens in Detroit and Traverse City and helped handicapped kids learn how to swim.

Besides working as a psychiatric physician's assistant, I'm also helping ovarian cancer patients and a couple of people with pancreatic cancer. I think it's an honor to assist somebody with cancer. That's the new paradigm—all us cancer patients helping each other and building association with each other. I'm writing a book called *Lifelines to the New World of Cancer Survival* to share what I know with other patients on a broader level.

The worst thing in the world is to worry and usurp your own power and give it to a medical center. Instead of playing around and doing guess work with chemo, my plan is to try to educate patients on how they can drive their own care. This new paradigm includes asking for molecular profiles, chemo sensitivity assays, and integrative medicine. The bottom line is to get patients to be more engaged, think outside of the box, and demand more personalized care. It's worked for me, and I believe it will work for others.

Lessons Learned

- Be in charge of your own health. It's not about the patients vs. the health care system; it's about saving your own life. Instead of going to the first oncologist you meet and starting treatment, step back and get at least two opinions or more. Don't be intimidated when a doctor says you need to hurry up and get treatment. That's not true unless you are critically ill or near death in the ICU. Most people have four or five weeks or more to get a second or third opinion. You need to look at the variety of options available and try not to get opinions from clinicians who work in the same medical center.

- Research possible targets for your tumor beyond the normal pathological/histological diagnosis your doctor gives you. For instance, for breast cancer, tests will show if the tumor is estrogen- and progesterone-positive or HER2-positive. This kind of histological pathology report is helpful in early-stage cancers, but not adequate for a more advanced cancer. You need more information, the kind you get from molecular profiles, to find a treatment that's targeted for your specific makeup of the tumor.

- Money should not be an issue when your life is at stake. Social workers, friends, family, and colleagues have helped me to raise money and get free treatment. Hospitals will help you if you ask them. And so will your friends and family. Organizations like Lend a Helping Hand can help organize fundraisers. You'd be surprised by the generosity of friends, relatives, and coworkers once you ask for help.

For more information about Mark, his work, and his upcoming book, Lifelines to the New World of Cancer Survival, *visit* www.cancercoachdrmark.com.

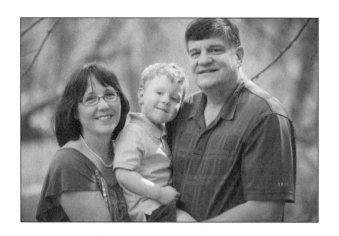

Don't Stop Believing

MARK WILLIAMS
Portland, OR
Age 57
Diagnosed in 2007 with stage IV melanoma

I was out on the river a lot growing up and didn't use sunscreen. My mom put cocoa butter on us and told us the darker you look, the better you are. That was the mindset in the '60s and early '70s. You'd never associate Oregon with melanoma, but we're one of the top five places in the country in melanoma diagnoses and top three in melanoma deaths. It is gray here a lot, and I think that's deceptive. Even if it's a cloudy day in the summer, the UV rays are more intense because the clouds filter out the good UV rays and let the bad ones through. There are a lot more tanning beds here, too, because it's so cloudy.

When I was diagnosed, I didn't have a mole. I just found a lump in my clavicle area. It was September 17, 2007, and we had just dropped our oldest daughter off to go to Europe for three months of college. I saw my general practitioner, and three days later I had a CT scan. She called me first thing in the morning and said I needed to get a biopsy. About a week and a half later, I had the surgery. That seemed like a quick progression to me. Nobody said let's wait a month.

After surgery, I was scheduled to visit with the ENT who performed it to discuss my results. I knew it was bad because they called me about six times, saying, "You have an appointment next week; are you going to make it?" They really wanted to make sure I was going to be there.

When I went to my appointment, I saw the nurse who was one of my customers at my flooring store. I knew her husband had cancer and asked how he was doing. She told me he died three years ago. It might have been a bad omen.

Sure enough, the doctor came in and said, "I have bad news; you have metastatic melanoma, and no one lives. You have no chance." I said, "No one?" He replied, "No, maybe one in a million. There are no treatments that will help you. You could try to get chemo, but it's not going to cure you; I guarantee it."

They took three lymph nodes out where I felt the lump; they were all tumors. He said, "I see one on your lung, but I'm not a lung specialist. It's wrapped around your collar bone and I couldn't cut them out. I have to send you right away to an oncologist."

Of course, I left there crushed. I went back to my office because my son was working there at the time. The saleswoman from the newspaper where I run ads was there and asked me what was wrong. When I told her she said, "Oh my God, my dad had that and he died in a month!" I said, "I'm going to get really sick now," and she turned white and walked out.

In the first two hours after my diagnosis, I was told no one lives and I'm going to die in a month. My brother took me out to eat and I cried throughout the meal. There was so much emotion going through my mind. Your whole world is spinning; you're reliving your kids' and your family's lives. It kept going through my mind, "My dad died in a month," and the doctor saying, "No one lives."

I went to work the next day and told my workers the news. It caught them off guard at first. They said they were going to quit and go to a place where the owner wasn't going to die. I said, "Just give me a couple of days to get my footing." They felt terrible about it and apologized the next day, but at the time, it was devastating.

My heart started pounding so I called up my brother and said, "Steve, can you come pick me up? I think I'm having a heart attack." He came over and we had a really good cry. There is a stigma that says grown men don't cry. Certainly that was the norm when I was raised, but it's totally false.

I settled down and then my heart started racing again, so he drove me to the hospital. If you want quick service, just say you're having a heart attack. They'll take you right away. When the emergency room doctor came in, I told him my story. He said, "I'm familiar with melanoma; my dad had it. Let's get a brain and chest scan and see what's going on."

He came back and said, "There's no cancer in your brain and none around your heart. I want you do this one thing for me: just take it one day at a time. Your job is to get through today and start tomorrow." He was really nice and told me his dad lived ten years with melanoma and I could too because they're always coming up with new therapies. That was at least an encouraging word and I started calming down.

I went to an oncologist, Dr. Yee, who performed a PET scan. On my fiftieth birthday, he called to tell me, "You have about fourteen tumors and a really big one on your esophagus—about nine by eight centimeters. There are nine tumors in your lungs and four more in your chest cavity. This is really bad. I normally don't do this over the phone, but that's what you asked."

My wife, Jan, threw me a surprise birthday party. Everybody brought framed pictures of me with them and reminisced. That was quite difficult because it was more of a wake than a birthday party. Everyone's heart was in the right place, but you have to get through that day and to the next one.

The next day we saw Dr. Yee, who referred me to Dr. Curti, a melanoma specialist at Providence Cancer Research Center who handles the toughest cases. Dr. Yee said, "Dr. Curti might have some trials for you; he has done this a long time and comes from the National Institute of Health (NIH)."

When we called Dr. Curti's office, they said we'd have to wait a month and a half for an appointment. I told them I couldn't wait, so he came in to see me on his day off. He sat me down and said, "Actually, there are options. We'll do a treatment called interleukin 2 (IL2), an immunotherapy which teaches the immune system to cure cancer. The downside is that it's a pretty intense treatment. We'll have to put you in the hospital, and you'll be very sick. I helped develop this clinical trial protocol at NIH, and I've done it a lot."

That's what you want—someone who knows how to handle the side effects and how to counteract it. When you looked online then, everything you saw said the only option was chemo, which really is the absolute worst thing you can do for melanoma. It shows little or no response. That was the first time I heard of immunotherapy.

I felt very confident with him, and that to me is always important. If you don't feel confident, you should find another doctor. It's still up to the patient to decide whether or not you do what they recommend. I felt confident he knew melanoma inside and out. It's a very tricky cancer; it doesn't really follow patterns.

Dr. Curti said, "I wish I could tell you it will never ever come back, but I can't." Rarely do doctors say they can cure cancer. When I was diagnosed, my goal was to make it to a month, and my next goal was make it to two months, and so on. As you survive longer, you start to gain a little confidence.

IL2 revs up your immune system, so you get fevers between 101–105 degrees. There were times I was sitting up talking normally and five seconds later, I was in full sweat and rigors. Minutes later I was so chilled I needed six blankets. Then I'd have a fever and headache for four hours. I had to change clothes every two hours.

The drug starts building up in your body after they give you more doses, then the symptoms last longer and longer. My skin flaked from head to toe nonstop, which lasted two to three years. It's one of the most intense treatments out there.

Each cycle required me to stay in the hospital for a week so they could monitor me and stop treatment if I was in a critical state. I wasn't allowed to leave unless I could prove I could urinate properly, walk, and eat solid foods. I went back to work within four days of leaving the hospital.

The first week I was in the hospital I was really angry that I had cancer and thought I didn't do anything to deserve it. I quickly changed my attitude and thought, *There's nothing easy about any of this, but they are doing what they need to make me better. You need to get in a calm mindset and concentrate on letting this agent do its job: Kill the cancer.*

The minute I learned I had cancer, I knew my life was never going to be the same. I told myself I'd have to do things that I thought I would never have to do, and that's the way it's got to be. The nurses encouraged me, saying, "You're going to feel pain in your chest. Try to think of it as little soldiers who are going to war with the cancer, and in any battle, there's going to be pain."

That first week I told Jan to go home at night to take care of our youngest daughter, who was sixteen. It's tough to spend seven days in a row in the hospital room. I hallucinated after my eighth dose of IL2, ripped my port out of my neck, and attempted to leave. (I don't recommend this.) After that week, my cousin came in to relieve Jan and stay from 11 p.m. to 7 a.m. every night. That helped a lot, just to know someone was there.

Dealing with cancer is tough on any sixteen-year-old (really the whole family), and my daughter was no different. She had many challenges, but unfortunately, we had so many other things we were worrying about. Looking back now, I probably would have handled things differently. We finally did tell our oldest daughter, who was in Europe studying, right before I started my treatment. We video chatted with her and set it up so she had two counselors there when we talked.

After a month of treatment, my doctor told us there was 50 percent shrinkage in my esophagus, the largest tumor. My lung tumors disappeared and the ones in my right chest were getting smaller as well. So I went back in for another cycle. As long as there is stable or shrinkage of tumors you are eligible to take up to six weeks of IL2.

In between cycles 4 and 5, we went to a Chinese restaurant while staying at our beach house in Newport with my brother, his kids, and wife. With our meal came the fortune cookies and the one I got said, "You are about to witness a miracle." At the time, I was pretty tired and didn't even think about it, but it was a sign of good things to come.

All in all, I had six weeks of treatments for a total of forty-eight doses. I finished my sixth week in April and had my next scan in June. It had been nine months since I was diagnosed with fourteen tumors. The scan was clear. Just as I was trying to wrap my head around that, in December, I went in for a routine scan. A lymph node came up in my chest that was positive for melanoma. I felt shot down, but my doctor said, "Don't freak out about this; it's just a bump in the road."

On January 9, 2009, which was my youngest daughter's eigtheenth birthday, I saw a surgeon who cut out fifty lymph nodes. The doctor recommended twenty-five rounds of radiation, which he said would kick-start the IL2 that was still in my system.

Melanoma is such a tricky animal and really aggressive. I've had friends say that in two weeks they've had eight tumors show up. So I had the radiation as soon as I recovered from the operation.

The radiologist told me I was strong enough to receive five times the normal dose, and I'd be done in five days. Business was slow, so I closed the shop down while I was getting it. I just put a sign on the door and came back to work when I was done.

I finished radiation in March 2009, and since then I've had no recurrences. All my scans have shown no cancer.

When I went into my last surgery, the anesthesiologist asked if I wanted music to play, so I requested "Don't Stop Believin'" by Journey. I think the song has a lot of meaning for cancer patients. There are times when you're lost. You truly are "living just to find emotion." It's helped to remind me to *not* stop believing. It works in life, as well.

My business is picking up, I feel good, and there are more people having positive results with melanoma treatments. We are making progress, but certainly not fast enough. There's still too many people dying. But we have to keep believing because what else do we have?

I tell people, "You never know what life is going to bring you." Out of all of our challenges, we have a beautiful grandson, Cashton, who we are raising. Sometimes you get a gift in surprising ways! It is unbelievably incredible that I can come home every night and have a little boy giving me a big hug and saying, "Papa, I love you!"

I feel incredibly blessed. We're super tired at the end of the day; I'm fifty-six and Jan is fifty-four. But it could be a lot worse. I go into Cashton's room every night and whisper in his ear "I love you," and Cashton whispers back, "I love you Papa. See you in the morning." It's an incredible experience that too many of my friends don't get to have.

We're just trying to be good people and carry it forward and encourage other people. When I was first diagnosed, I couldn't find anyone who had survived. I told the people at the hospital in Providence that if I could do anything to help spread awareness or mentor patients through treatment, to let me know. It is a scary road. If you can meet people who have been through it and give an encouraging word, that's exactly what we need. And what I do.

Social media has been a godsend. There is a page called "Bad Ass Melanoma Warriors" that was started by a stage III survivor in Missouri. Through this group, many melanoma survivors of all stages got together in North Carolina for a melanoma research fundraising event through a foundation called Aim@Melanoma. We are bringing Cashton this year and taking him to the Nascar Hall of Fame. I also participate in the Portland AIM@Melanoma walk, and I'm on the Leadership Board of Directors at Providence Cancer Center. I'm here today because of Providence and how they were able to manage my side effects, and remind me to "Don't Stop Believin'." I'm one of the few people who were able to work through their IL2 treatments.

Everybody handles it differently, but I can't just say I had cancer, and it's no big deal. I lose a friend a month; I know it's a big deal. It's a life-changing experience. There are only about one thousand people in the world who have lived as long as I have with stage IV metastatic melanoma. But this number will increase because of places like Providence Cancer Center. I know I'm very, very blessed.

Lessons Learned

- Live one day at a time.
- Every day is truly a gift.
- Don't stop believing. You have to keep moving forward. If you hit a roadblock during one treatment, try a second. Don't give up the first sign something's not working. Try to find a Plan B, C, and D.

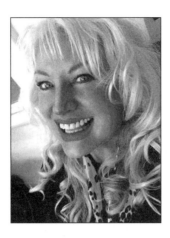

Becoming Friends with My Cancer

NANCY SIMPSON
Cincinnati, OH
Age 62
Living with stage IV lymphocytic leukemia since 2005

I was a codependent people-pleaser all my life. I stayed in my first marriage too long because I wanted to do the right thing. I did the same thing in my second marriage, being way too nice in a difficult situation. I was always happy, breezy, and fun, so people liked me, and that made me feel good.

When I was diagnosed, I was working in a prison as a therapist for violent male repeat felons—murderers and rapists. I quickly learned that I had to become an alpha dog—tough and dominant. It wasn't easy, but with those men, you had to go toe-to-toe, stare them down, and channel your strongest, toughest person. I quickly morphed into a person that I had never been—a strong woman who could control powerful men. The experience helped me to get in touch with my power, which I believe helped me along my cancer journey.

I had absolutely no symptoms other than a lump on my neck, but it wasn't bothering me. I happened to mention it to my oldest child, Erin, who encouraged me to tell my doctor the next time I saw her. When I went for my visit, she said, "This doesn't really feel like anything to me, but we'll keep a watch on it." The next time I saw the doctor, about six months later, the lump was still there, so she recommended an anti-biotic. It still didn't go away.

Erin said, "That's ridiculous! It's been eight months! Your doctor's an idiot; you need an appointment with mine." I didn't want to go to a new doctor, but she insisted, so I went. When I went to see her doctor, she said, "It doesn't feel like anything, but let's make Erin happy and get a CT scan."

The CT scan came back as suspicious for reactive node disease or leukemia or lymphoma. She told me I needed to go to the hospital and get a biopsy. So I went. When the surgeon walked in the room after my procedure, I knew it was cancer. He didn't have to say anything. Because he was a general surgeon, he said he couldn't tell me anything other than it was leukemia.

So I went to the oncologist who actually said these words to me, "How interesting. You have one of the last truly incurable cancers." Astonished, I said, "Are you telling me that I'm dying?" He just responded that we're all dying, until I demanded the truth. He finally said, "You have a fatal disease."

In that moment, my complete world turned upside down. I told myself I was dead. I walked out of his office, a zombie, a dead woman walking. Everything was gray; there was no more color. When I went out, I saw all these people who were alive; they had a future. I didn't care about clothes, purses, kids, or anything. I would wake up in the middle of the night, and I would be normal Nancy; then all of a sudden the thought would hit me, *You're dying; you have an incurable leukemia.*

I had been divorced for six years at that point, so I was all by myself. There was no person to hold onto, nobody to tell how scared I was.

I began to see my leukemia as an army of worms that were eating me alive and were growing and growing. I was mental.

Both of my ex-husbands were very wealthy, and I was used to living in palatial splendor. I went from being financially secure to facing poverty. I left my job, and my COBRA was $700 a month. I had to wait twenty-four months to get on early Medicare and during that wait period, I had to pay 20 percent of my medical bills. It totally wiped me out. When I finally got on disability, I only received $1,200 a month, and that was taxed. The good news was I had hit poverty level and qualified to receive help from the Leukemia/Lymphoma Society. They helped me with my medical bills to the tune of $500 a month for two years. They completely saved me because my kids were all in college and didn't have money like that to help me.

About three months after my diagnosis, I went to church where the minister was giving a sermon saying, "There is no divorce, there's no bankruptcy, no valley, no depth of being, no place the faith of God is not." And I believe that in that moment, apart from my own self, a miracle of grace happened to me. I believed every single leukemic cell was transformed into the shining, radiant face of God. I looked around the room, and no longer was I dying; I was alive again. I was not focused on my death, but on the fact I was alive and that God was inside of me.

And a couple of weeks after that I was thinking about love and grace and forgiveness, and I said to my leukemia, "I just want you to know that I forgive you. I really forgive you." And my leukemia, I felt, spoke to me and said, "Nancy, we do not want to hurt you. We don't know how to get better. We don't know how to stop dividing. We love you, and we feel so sorry that we can't. We don't want to be leukemia cells; we want to be happy, healthy cells. Do everything you can to heal us. Eat right, exercise, and take chemo if you need it, but we want to work with you so we can all get better."

At that point, I became friends with my leukemia and started working together with it. Ever since that day, me and my leukemia have been working to stay well and heal.

At first, I refused to do chemo because my paradigm was chemo is poison. I had always eaten whole, organic foods. Why would a sick person further hurt their body by ingesting poison? I did high colonics and every supplement known to man and read Louise Hay and everything else about healing your body through your thoughts. But I was getting sicker and sicker. The leukemia affected my eyes, and I began to go blind. I had big prisms in my glasses and if I took them off, I could not see a person's face. Everything was a blur.

And my neutrophil (a type of white blood cell) count kept dropping, putting me at a high risk for infection. If it's fewer than five hundred, you can get an infection and die. My neutrophil count stayed at about two hundred for about two years. The oncologists kept telling me I had to do chemo, but I still believed chemo was so awful.

In 2011, I went for a doctor visit and my cell count was at zero. She said, "Okay, honey, if I send you out and you get pneumonia, you'll die; you're at death's doorstep. You want to die, you can die." I was crying, and I said, "I don't want to die."

I started my first chemo that day, and since then I've been going every twelve weeks for a six-hour infusion. I've been on several different treatments and right now I am on Rituxan.

Because of the chemo and leukemia, my main symptoms are extreme fatigue and muscle and bone pain. If it gets too bad, I have narcotics, but I don't like to use them. I tend to transcend the pain by just thinking, *You are so lucky you can walk and see. You are so lucky you're not in hospice and you have your own home.* Sometimes it feels like climbing Mt. Everest just doing little things like housework, but I tell myself I can do it and use it as a challenge. And I have such a sense of accomplishment when I'm done. I'm like, *Yes girl, you did it!*

Every single day I try to look cute and get out of the house, even if it's just to the grocery store. I try to go to my favorite coffee shop every day. I call it "my office." All my friends will say, "Did you go to your office today?" And I'm also blessed that I know a lot of people who take me to cool places during the week. Each time is a holy adventure to me, even if it's just to a coffee shop.

This past summer, they had free yoga at a local park every Tuesday night, which attracted about three to four hundred people each time. I could barely move, so it was kind of intimidating, but I figured there were hundreds of people and no one would see me. In the beginning, I had to stop and rest, and I couldn't do everything they did, but just trying made me feel so empowered. And I went every single Tuesday night for three months. By the end of the summer, I could do just about everything for that whole hour. It made me so proud that I could stretch my body and make my body go into the downward dog and child's poses. There are no words to tell you how wondrous that experience was to me.

I was mostly in pain, but they say you're supposed to talk to your body. So I said to the pain, "Hey, we're doing this." I still do yoga. I have a laptop and do yoga stretches, along with people on YouTube. I put the laptop on my bed, and I do yoga with people who are in the mountains, the beach, and in really cool studios.

I get such a sense of accomplishment challenging myself. Right now I'm training to walk in the Flying Pig Marathon here in Cincinnati. It's surreal to think I'm hanging out with runners and planning to do this. Last night I walked a nineteen-minute mile. I am the slowest one in the group, but I'm doing it!

I eat virtually no processed foods. I find it interesting that with my limited finances, I can actually eat better for less. Vegetables just aren't that expensive, especially when they're from people's gardens in the summer.

For my well-being, I try to keep away from negative people and from my own negative thoughts if they come. I hear them, but I don't dwell on them; I try to let them pass through me.

I feel like I have to have a purpose for living. I don't want to be just sucking in the air and not giving back. Every single day, I wake up and I ask the universe to use me to help lighten the load of someone on the earth. So when I go to the grocery store, I find people who look sad and smile at them and try to get them to smile back. Or give a real compliment. I try to lift the load. And when I go to my coffee shop, there's always poor people walking around on the street. I look them in the eye and say "Hi, how are you?" And on Facebook, every single day I write one cheery, positive thing and give positive words of hope and encouragement. And then I feel like I've done a good thing; I've been a value to the world that day.

I'm so lucky to have wonderful friends who help me. The hardest thing for me is being alone. I'm on disability, which means I'm financially challenged. One friend bought me $20 gift cards for my coffee shop, and I thought I had won the Mega Millions lottery. Another friend took me to Whole Foods Market and told me to fill a shopping cart, and she paid for it. These are little things, but to me, they are so big! I have all I really need and then some. I may not have massive funds, but I live an incredible life of splendor.

I'm a grandma now to Alice, who is three, and Hazel, who is five months old. Every moment with them is holy; it's magic. I can't even believe I get to be with them. Every once in a while I get this tinge of, "I never want to not be here." I don't want this little family to ever go on without me in it. I always want to be with my family. I want to be with these precious little girls and watch them grown up. But I know that everybody has these feelings ... we all get old and die.

I hold a cup of coffee in my hand and I'm like, "Wow, I'm in a coffee shop, able to hold a cup of coffee, and it smells good. I'm so grateful." I get in my car, and I'm so grateful I have money for gas and it can take me places. I'm so grateful I have my own little house, and it's mine. I'm just so full of gratitude. I don't think I would be this way to the extent I am without the lesson cancer has afforded me.

Lessons Learned

- Explore the idea of working with your disease and not fighting against it. What would it look like if we work with the cancer to get well?

- Explore cancer organizations' benefits, especially those dedicated to your particular type of cancer.
- Consider joining online support groups. They have been awesome for me. I have friends all over the country who I met through my groups. I never met them in real life, but feel like I know them. Groups like the Lighthouse Leukemia Support Facebook group nourished me and gave me love.

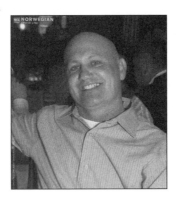

Getting in the Ring with Cancer

PETER DEVEREAUX
Boston, MA
Age 50
Living with stage IV, HER2-positive breast cancer since 2008

In high school, I started getting into boxing and running. I never looked forward to a fight in the street, but I really loved to box. About 98 percent of the people were great and loving. But there were some who were tough punks and dealt drugs. I didn't have to fight very much, but I was confident in a quiet way. I didn't worry because I knew I could handle myself.

I realized later in my life that I was meant to box. It helped bring down my stress level. If I got angry, I could always hit the bag. It was one of the things that kept me in balance because I was a very energetic kid. Years later, my brother Joe and I trained hard and got into the Golden Gloves tournament, which is how you make it into the Olympics. We both did very well, but didn't make it. We were in phenomenal shape, though. You can't get a better workout than boxing.

As I approached graduation, I listened to my friends plans for the future. College wasn't as strong an option as it is now. I didn't want to hang around and do a meaningless job. My dad is my idol; he was in the Marines. I thought, *This guy is a real man.* My dad is going to be eighty-three next month, and he's still the man. I wanted to make something of my life and I loved being an American, so I joined. By far, the job I'm most proud of is representing my country and being a Marine.

When you're eighteen years old and you're a Marine, you become a man in a heartbeat. People talk about stress in a job; if you want to know stress, become a Marine. If you mess up in your job, you could kill one of your fellow Marines. It was a good life lesson. I learned how to deal with all types of people and situations and that you have to be dependent on each other. Overall, I'm definitely a better man for going into the Marines. Ironically, the job I'm most proud of is the job that gave me breast cancer.

I was diagnosed on January 11, 2008. My daughter Jackie was ten at the time. I was working as a machinist full-time and part-time as a landscaper on some nights and weekends. My wife, Fiona, was and still is working as a recruiter.

When I woke up for work on Friday morning at 4 a.m., I got out of bed and my hand bumped into my chest. I noticed a lump. I thought it was fatty tissue, since I was forty-five and wasn't working out as hard as I used to. I was playing in a few basketball leagues, so I also thought I might have gotten bumped in the chest. Guys are horrible about going to the doctor. At least I made an appointment.

With male breast cancer, even if you go to a doctor, they usually don't know anything about it, so they ignore it. My doctor, though, took immediate action and ordered a mammogram and ultrasound. The next day I had a core biopsy. The day after that, they called and said I had breast cancer.

Of course it's shocking to be diagnosed with any kind of cancer, but, as a dude, it's especially shocking to have what a lot of people consider to be a women's disease. I was looking in the other room and Jackie was watching "SpongeBob" and I was thinking how I would tell her. The first thing I thought is that I had to be there for my daughter. I didn't know if I was going to cry or scream.

Fiona had to work late, so she wasn't going to be home until 7 or 8 p.m. I called and told her, "I have to tell you something, but I can't tell you over the phone." I ended up having to tell her over the phone anyway. She came home early from work, of course, and said, "Let's see what we're going to do next and develop an action plan."

We told our daughter, and it broke my heart. Fiona's mother got breast cancer when she was seventy-two, and like with many older women, the cancer was more slow-growing and not as aggressive. She had great results; her hair came back softer and really nice. She looked good and came back strong. Basically I told Jackie that her grandmother had it, so hopefully I'll get through like her grandma, too. It was still tough, but at least we had a good example we could use. Jackie just said, "okay."

Fiona was so supportive. We were both scared. As a guy, I was so uneducated. It seemed like there were two types of breast cancer: the kind they can cure and the kind that is fatal. I wondered which kind I had. We had to put on a front for Jackie like everything was alright while we were gathering so much information. We took it one step at a time.

The next day we had to do a bone scan and chest X-ray. We received the results the next day. I had surgery on January 18, 2008. They ended up taking out twenty-two lymph nodes and they were all cancerous. I was diagnosed with stage IIIB breast cancer.

In February, I started my first chemo. I had a thirteen-month program, which consisted of twenty-nine treatments and thirty radiation appointments. I was on a clinical trial taking Lapatinib and Tykerb at the same time. My chemo was scheduled to end April 9, 2009. A few days before that, I started to get shooting pains down my spine. I contacted my doctors.

When I came in on my scheduled last appointment, we did scans. We found out the cancer had traveled to my spine, ribs, and hip. I felt so much rage. The treatment kicked my butt from the jump. I wondered if the treatment worked at all. But I knew I better learn more about metastatic cancer. I started on a new treatment and I've never been off of it since.

Dana Farber is phenomenal. Right after we left our appointment, we saw a social worker. We had a great relationship with her. We asked, "How do we come home and tell our daughter and others that my cancer spread?" They helped us with everything.

Several months later in August 2008, I received a letter from the Marines stating that while I was at Camp Lejeune (from 1980 to 1984), I might have come in contact with contaminated water. At that point, they had no idea I had breast cancer, but this letter went out supposedly to all Marines who were stationed there. Not every man and woman received a letter. It literally took an act of Congress just to send out that paperwork.

I'll never forget, it was on a Wednesday when I received the letter. When I got it, boom, instantly a light went off and I thought, *There's no doubt this was the cause.*

We filled out the paperwork called the Water Registry Report, then found a website called "The Few, The Proud, The Forgotten" for people affected by the contamination. Once we got on the site, Mike Partain instant-messaged me and gave me his number. Mike was born on the base while his father was in the service. He was keeping count of how many people contracted cancer. We talked on the phone and started to put the puzzle together.

Camp Lejeune is huge; it's a self-contained city and everyone used the same water source. The Marines were dumping toxins into that water over a thirty-year period. Basically, there were three different ways the water was contaminated. One was dry cleaning solvents (TCE). Everything was dry cleaned on the base; you never see a Marine with a wrinkly uniform. The other culprit was degreasers (PCE) from cleaning all the engines of vehicles. The third thing was benzene, which is gasoline.

Gasoline is one of the contaminants the Marines hid over the years; all the others were public record. It was estimated that 800,000 to 1.2 million gallons of gasoline were dumped into the drinking water. It's indisputable. The water always got tested and reports concluded the compounds were two to four hundred times the legal limit, and nothing was done.

Since I received that letter, it's been a non-stop journey. I've spoken a few times at Congressional hearings. Almost every member of *The Few, The Proud, The Forgotten* makes it their main goal to prevent this from happening ever again. It's beyond criminal; so many lives were lost.

I was one of the first guys in the country to get benefits for male breast cancer due to the water contamination at Camp Lejeune. There are eighty-three of us now. It's the largest male breast cancer cluster ever recorded. The male breast cancer cases drew the most attention, but unfortunately there are about seven other types of cancers, still-born babies, and birth defects that are associated with it. You go to the cemetery on the base, and 25 percent of babies didn't make it because of the water contamination.

Camp Lejeune is not the only base that's been contaminated, but it's the worst ever recorded. They came out with an Emmy-nominated documentary called *Semper Fi* on the journey of this whole situation. The film briefly shows a photo shoot for our group's 2010 male breast cancer calendar. The calendar, which raised awareness about male breast cancer, featured thirteen of us from Camp Lejeune from all over the country. It also raised money for research into the environmental causes of breast cancer.

The documentary is really about one unbelievable American, Jerry Ensminger. Jerry was a drill instructor who lost his daughter to childhood leukemia. He's really the person who started exposing the contamination's link to cancer. He was the only one who was going to DC to get answers. They already had the ball rolling and had done the hard work when I came along. I just spoke to Congress a few times.

If you're part of the government, you can't sue the government. If the Marines were a private industry, their leaders would be in prison all of their lives. That's one of the disheartening things. It took them so long and really they're not admitting they're 100 percent at fault. We drank water by the gallons; we chugged it because we were training all the time.

They say, "You never leave a fallen soldier behind," and Marines take care of their own. They haven't lived by their own values. We've had to beg and fight for everything. Finally, a law passed called The Janey Ensminger Act, which made sure the Marines affected by the Camp Lejeune contamination had health benefits. It was named after Jerry's daughter. This law will take care of those who don't have benefits. I was the one who carried the benefits for my family, but when I could no longer work, we were covered under Fiona's benefits. A lot of guys didn't have that option.

It pisses me off that I was so proud of being a Marine and I have to fight them now. None of us like it, but we have to. They were ignorant and thought we'd be fine. If they could rewind the tape and go back, I'm sure they would.

At one point, I was writing a book about my journey, but stopped writing after my recurrence. I'm in the process of starting back. In my book, I want to tell what it's like to be the only dude in the room: most rooms you're in related to breast cancer, you are the only dude. My whole life, I've been surrounded by dudes. I was in the Marines, then I worked in construction. Most of the time, I wish there was a different reason than having breast cancer to be surrounded by women.

Honestly, it's a great thing. I always knew women were prettier and smarter. I always thought men were tougher and stronger, but this breast cancer experience has taught me we don't even have that over women.

Women are naturally more compassionate. Initially I felt kind of weird being around so many women, but once I asked for help, I was accepted without question. I said, "I'm on the team. I'll wear pink or whatever you want, but give me some scoop on what's going on here." I've never had a bad experience. The great thing about women is you ask for help, and they'll give it.

I recently went to a Metastatic Breast Cancer Network (MBCN) conference and met two other dudes who were survivors. And that's a lot of guys. Most guys aren't at these conferences. You can go up to a woman and just ask them questions without knowing them. They know you aren't there to pick them up. The pick-up line at a breast cancer conference is, "Hey what treatment are you on?" It's a welcoming crew. We're not sneaking out of this disease, so let's enjoy the ride. I feel very honored to connect with so many spectacular women.

I've learned a lot at conferences and met a lot of patient advocates. Just talking with them, you find out a lot. When I first was diagnosed, I felt like there were no other men out there. Now I try to be that guy for them to talk to. I try to be an educated advocate, so I can respond when people ask me questions.

At the MBCN conference, I learned that anytime your cancer travels to a different spot, if possible, you should do a biopsy and have the tumor tested to see if your cancer has changed. I've never heard that before. My cancer just traveled to the lining of my liver, so it's something I'll bring up to my doctor.

I've been through eleven treatments. I finally started writing this stuff down and find out how many more treatments are available for my type of cancer. We're looking for a treatment for the long run. So far, my current treatment, Gemcitabine, is doing well. My tumor markers have gone down tremendously. The treatment is taking a beating on my white blood cells and platelets. Sometimes I'll get blood work and they'll tell me I can't get treatment that day, but I can do the Herceptin every three weeks (which I've been doing on and off for five years).

I also take Zometa for my bones. After five years, it can make your bones brittle. I knew a woman who was on it whose leg suddenly shattered while she was taking a walk. So I had a discussion with my doctor to ask about other options. Two years ago, I went from getting it once a month, to getting it every three or four months. Now I do it twice a year and take a supplement to keep my bones strong. I'm trying to be proactive rather than wait.

I'm into integrative medicine. I think you need chemotherapy, but I don't think that's enough. I just look at how initially I was only on chemotherapy, and the cancer spread. So I look for other things I can do so my body can receive these toxins to get rid of cancer.

When I was an athlete, I juiced a lot. My wife and I have been juicing. I'm also researching supplements and taking mushrooms in a pill form because they help with your white blood cells. I tell my oncologist everything, but they just don't know about supplements. For me, mentally, I'm taking a mushroom that's all natural and is the highest quality you can find. It's just another little thing I'm doing.

At times, I'm juicing every day; then I slack off for a while. You still have to be human. I eat a lot of fruits and vegetables. Once a month if I want a food and it's not on my preferred list, I'll just eat it. Burgers are my thing. I'm a cheap date. Sometimes you just feel like living. About 80 percent of the time I follow a plan. That works for me. I don't want to live always denying myself.

I'm doing well. My goal right now is that I get to the point when they say NED—No Evidence of Disease. Enough of it already! You ride the roller coaster. Sometimes you go through a treatment that doesn't work, then you find a treatment that's working. I'm trying to stay healthy by eating and sleeping well, exercising, and not stressing too much. I'm doing well, and want to keep it going a long time.

This year, Dana Farber's Jimmy Fund celebrated the sixtieth anniversary of its fundraising telethon. The Red Sox players often come and visit patients at the Jimmy Fund unit at Dana Farber. I was nominated to be one of the cancer patients and they invited me and my family to the game. It was a Friday night game with the Yankees, our big rival. I don't care what age you are; I stood on that mound to throw the first pitch, and I was like a thirteen-year-old kid. Unfortunately we lost the game, and the joke was they should have kept me in a couple of innings; I'd do better.

Moments like that I'll never forget. There's nothing like being at Fenway Park to watch the Red Sox. As great as that was, meeting my wife Fiona and having our daughter Jackie were the happiest times of my life. I'd never really loved a girl before Fiona. I always loved and respected women; I was brought up like that. But Fiona was the first woman I really loved. When I finally met her and got married and had a child—that outweighed anything else I've accomplished.

Having cancer has changed my relationship with my family. I used to be the one who got everything done; now I'm the one getting things done for me. I'm one of the richest guys I know, not financially, but because of the love and support and good energy I have around me. I'm so fortunate. I have all these siblings, nephews, and nieces . . . they've all been there for me. We have all changed for the better.

I use the analogy of going into the ring with cancer. It's definitely the toughest opponent I've had. I never thought when I was fighting these tough guys that later on I'd be in the fight for my life. Everything I've gone through has prepared me for where I am today.

Lessons Learned

- Whether you're a man or a woman, you need to check yourself. Women know their bodies; men aren't as in tune with their bodies as they should be. If you notice something wrong like nipple discharge, an inverted nipple, or a lump in your chest, get it checked out. Don't wait.
- If you're not satisfied with your treatment, always get a second opinion and a third opinion, if needed.
- Don't wait until you get a life-threatening disease to be present and appreciate life. I used to hear all these corny sayings like,

"Appreciate the little things because you find out later in life that the little things are the big things." It wasn't until I was diagnosed metastatic that I realized that's true.

- Having a positive attitude helps you appreciate more things in life.
- Be nice to yourself and other people, and you'll be surprised what it brings to you.

A note from the author: I am very sad to report that Peter passed away on August 20, 2014. He was a fighter until the end, an inspiration to many and a loving husband, father, and friend. It is our hope that sharing his story will help ensure his legacy will live on.

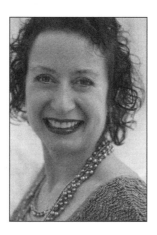

A Rare Calling

SUSAN THORNTON
Philadelphia, PA
Age 55
Diagnosed in 1991 with advanced cutaneous lymphoma

I spent twenty-eight years of my career in healthcare information technology. I feel lucky that I have a little insight into the healthcare arena from the business side, but it doesn't always help you when you become a patient. That's a whole different kettle of fish, as they say.

In 1989, I got my dream job with the number one healthcare software company at the time and moved back to the Philadelphia area from Colorado. Then I discovered an annoying, itchy rash around my waist that didn't go away. I went to different dermatologists over the course of about a year and a half. They gave me all different kinds of lotions and potions to try to make it go away, but nothing ever seemed to work.

Finally, a friend referred me to a dermatologist who had helped her with a really bad spider bite. I made an appointment to go during my lunch hour. After looking at it, she called in her colleague and took my history. She said, "I'm going to do a biopsy, but I'm pretty certain that you have a rare form of cancer called mycosis fungoides (a form of cutaneous T-cell lymphoma). I'm going to send you down to an expert in Philadelphia."

That really wasn't what I thought I was going to hear when I walked into the dermatologist's office that day. I went back to my office, gathered up my stuff, and told my administrative person I had just been diagnosed with a rare form of cancer and I had to go see my mother.

It came out of the blue. I just had this little rash. How could that possibly be anything but dermatitis, eczema? That's what everyone was telling me it was. Now all of a sudden it morphed into this rare form of cancer that sounded like a weird fungus.

We went to see Dr. Eric Vonderheid in Philadelphia who was one of just a handful of experts in this particular field. Still today, it's a very rare form of lymphoma. I remember he was a very grandfatherly type of gentleman and very kind and compassionate.

We were sitting in front of him and he said, "Well, you know, it's a very rare disease, but we can treat it. In rare cases, it becomes aggressive, but for most people, that doesn't happen. I fully expect that we will be able to manage this, although there's no cure. The typical patient is an African-American male over sixty, and you don't quite fit the profile. But we can manage this."

Because it's not curable and mostly chronic, I started with photo-chemotherapy (PUVA). I took a chemotherapy drug called Psoralen, which photosynthesizes the skin, and stood in a light box for a few minutes. The interaction of the light and the photosensitivity of your skin impacts the malignant T-cells and kills them.

So I did that for three months, and they were gracious enough to work around my busy schedule. It wasn't bad; you basically get a tan, so I looked really healthy. I had to wear big, funky goggles for twenty-four hours because the photosensitivity makes your eyes very sensitive to the light. My boss nicknamed me Suzy Sprocket. I didn't tell too many people. The rash faded away after three months, so I was like, "Great; I'm done! Good deal!" But unfortunately for me, that didn't really last.

I did a couple of rounds of PUVA for the first few years, and that seemed to work okay. Then unfortunately, I became one of the five to ten percent of people whose disease becomes aggressive and just doesn't really react well to the treatment.

We started adding interferon injections, trying to bolster my immune system. Then I tried some other topical chemotherapy agents, such as nitrogen mustard. But then the supply ran out, so I had to try something else. My disease continued to progress; I had more lesions on my body that were thicker and very, very itchy. I started to get them on my neck and on my face so they became very visible, which is also a challenging part of this disease.

The itching was so intolerable; I didn't sleep for many years. Unless you've experienced it, it's really hard to describe. I had shooting pain, and it felt like ants were crawling out of my body. There's nothing that can stop the itch. I tried cold compresses, oatmeal baths, and every lotion I could find. Nothing works except getting your disease under control.

I was on one therapy that had just been FDA-approved, but it threw off my hormones so much that I was a basket case. Most people who get diagnosed with this disease are older. I was in my thirties and pre-menopausal.

At one point, my copay was around $1,800 a month. I was a single woman, trying to pay my mortgage and keep my job. I needed my insurance, and it's a scary place to be when you start looking at that kind of money. No one ever plans to be ill, but especially when you're in your thirties, who thinks you're going to have this financial impact?

I tried to not dwell on it and just kept doing what I needed to do. I think doing something physical really helped me get through some of the darkest hours. I had been a runner for a long time, and I contin-ued to run even when I was really sick. I think that was something that I could hold on to and have control over.

I also did a lot of research on diet and other kinds of holistic treatments and started doing meditation and energy work.

By 1998, my disease had gone into full-blown tumor stage. I had patches and weepy tumors all over my body. My whole face was red and crusty, and I had a tumor under my chin. I had tumors in my scalp and my right eye was closed because of a tumor. They reeked, and it was just ugly.

It was pretty scary to look at myself in the mirror most days when I was in bad shape. I did my best to cover up with makeup. I had to wash my hair a couple of times a day because of the weepy tumors on my scalp.

I was fortunate I had a flexible job. I was in sales, so I wasn't always in the office. I could go to an appointment and go back to the hotel room and wash my hair and reapply makeup. It was still hard. I saw a psychologist and had support from family, which helped. I've always kept a journal, and I think writing about it when I was really in the depth of despair and fear also helped me. I had a lot of dialogue with God in the middle of the night when I woke up in tears because of scratching so much. Everything was bleeding because of that.

That spring, I couldn't go on anymore. My doctor told me my disease was life-threatening and my only option was a stem cell transplant. If I didn't go down that road, I wouldn't be here; the disease would just take over. I was only thirty-nine years old and would have to be out of work for at least a year. I was in total panic.

There was a turning point for me when I knew that if I didn't do something drastic, I was going to die. I had a true burning desire to live no matter what. I had to do whatever I needed to make sure that I could stay on the planet.

So we began the process for the stem cell transplant and in preparation, I had to start going through all the tests and find a donor. It had to be a match and, back in 1998, there wasn't a big database of donors. But even before I got to that point, they had to get the disease under control. So I began on doses of prednisone and started targeted electron beam radiation. The radiation to my head caused me to lose all my hair, but it eventually grew back. I had to get radiation every day and used up all of my vacation time, so I took a medical leave of absence.

It was fascinating to me that there were some people who couldn't be with me because I officially looked like a cancer patient with no hair, eyebrows, or eyelashes. But I was blessed with some amazing friends and family members who really rallied around me and supported me no matter how horrible I looked.

I received great news when I was done with all of my radiation in September: I didn't need the stem cell transplant! I had one really large lymph node that they took out. They thought they would find a lot of the cancer, but there wasn't a lot in there. So luckily for me, the disease didn't get beyond the skin. I turned forty that September and threw myself a huge birthday party to celebrate.

My physicians were really amazed I didn't ultimately need the stem cell transplant. I don't think they know why. Divine intervention, perhaps? I can't really explain it. I should have gone down that road, but then I didn't have to.

Throughout my treatment, I had an inner knowing that there was a reason for me to go through this process. In 2001, I decided I wanted to give back because I felt very lucky. I signed up for my first triathlon to raise money for the Leukemia and Lymphoma Society. I have been hooked on triathlons since.

After that, I got really engaged with my local chapter of the Leukemia and Lymphoma Society. I became a triathlon coach, then was asked to sit on the board of directors for the local chapter.

In 2008, my oncologist retired, and I had to find a new one. I went to Dr. Lessin, who was one of the cofounders of the Cutaneous Lymphoma Foundation. During my first appointment, he recruited me to come and check out the board. Eventually, I resigned from the Leukemia and Lymphoma Foundation board and joined the Cutaneous Lymphoma Foundation's board. I thought, "Oh gosh, why hadn't I done this before? It's my disease. I could give back directly."

I became more involved and in 2011, I quit my corporate job to manage the foundation's programs and services. A year later, the executive director resigned and I was asked if I would come onboard and take the leadership position.

The Cutaneous Lymphoma Foundation is a non-profit patient advocacy organization dedicated to supporting every person with cutaneous lymphoma by promoting awareness and education, advancing patient care, and facilitating research.

It's a rare disease; we estimate there are only thirty thousand people who have been diagnosed in North America. The incidence is somewhere around two to three thousand new diagnoses a year. But it's often misdiagnosed as eczema, psoriasis, or dermatitis and may not be diagnosed for five to seven years.

Because of this, it can be very isolating and, very frightening. It's hard to find an oncologist or dermatologist who is familiar with the disease and other people who are dealing with it.

We support people all over the world, teaching them about cutaneous lymphoma and allowing them to support and connect with others. We do eight annual full-day events around the country every year. We'll be doing our first event in Montreal this summer, and we're doing some collaboration with physicians in the United Kingdom. If people can't get to our live programs, they can go online to watch the videos and hear from the experts in the field.

Because cutaneous lymphoma is very visible, there's the whole emotional element to living with it. I am still living with it, although it has gotten much better. I still have a couple of little spots, including one on my neck.

I was at the train station in Washington DC this weekend and the guy behind the counter said to me, "Oh, is that a hickey on your neck?" I laughed and said, "Oh, yes, I should be so lucky! No, it's cancer." I've learned to have a sense of humor because you just don't know what people are going to say.

In retrospect, I think I couldn't be in a position I'm in today as the CEO of the Cutaneous Lymphoma Foundation had I not went through the emotional, physical, and financial impact of this cancer.

I'm learning how to be vulnerable. I was brought up in a culture that taught you to suck it up. You take the hard stuff, and you don't whine about it. It was really hard to open up and share my inner fears. I didn't want to burden anyone with my disease or how I felt. So I kept a lot of things really close to the vest.

Now I get to share my story with other people who are going through this disease and hopefully give them hope and inspiration that they can live with it and have a good life.

Most people never meet anyone else with cutaneous lymphoma. Being able to talk to someone who has been down the road and come out the other side is so helpful. You get to build these personal relationships with people. It's totally amazing. We did our first ever two-day patient conference last June, which really gave people an opportunity to interact with fellow patients and physicians. It was just magical.

One woman came up to me, grabbed me by the hands, and said, "I just can't thank you enough. You saved my life." I always am speechless when people say that because to me, I'm just providing insight or ideas, or sharing my experience.

I feel like the luckiest person on this planet. I often say to people, "Who gets to work every day with other people and patients who have your same disease?" I get to interact with experts all around the world and hear the latest and greatest research on this small rare disease.

If you had told me even ten years ago that I would be here doing this work and have it be my full-time job, I would have said you're out of your mind. But here I am, and I feel so fortunate.

Lessons Learned

- Listen to your inner voice. One of the big challenges for so many people is getting to the right clinicians. I think physicians and researchers are brilliant and wonderful, but they don't always know everything. I believe every human being has their own innate guidance system. A lot of times, we don't listen to it because we think we don't know enough, but it's really important when you have decisions to make.

- Educate yourself about your disease. If something doesn't feel right, stand up for what you feel is the best for you. But it's important that you are coming from a place of knowledge.

- Surround yourself with supportive, positive people. Even if they may not always agree with your perspective, they should honor it. I've learned to surround myself with people who are my cheerleaders and supporters versus the doubters who always see things from a negative perspective.

For more information about the Cutaneous Lymphoma Foundation, go to www.clfoundation.org.

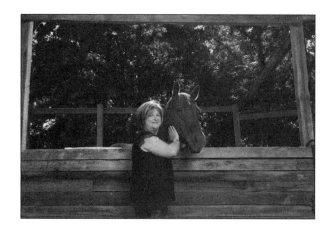

Writing Hope in the Sand

SUZANNE LINDLEY
Canton, TX
Age 46
Living with stage IV colon cancer since 1998

My dad was disabled in Vietnam. He had a skull fracture, and when he came back, he didn't remember my mom and didn't know how to walk and talk. When I was four, he and I learned how to read together. He could not go back to work, so he was "Mr. Mom." My mom worked at a library, so my dad would take me to school every day, and as I got older, would fix lunch when I walked home from school.

I saw my dad go through things I cannot even imagine, and he never, ever complained. He had his health challenges as I was growing up, but he had amazing strength. He learned to walk, talk, and do other things people predicted were impossible. Everything he did was a miracle.

When I was eighteen, his liver began to fail from non-A, non-B hepatitis. They said he contracted it from blood transfusions he received in Vietnam. I think Agent Orange may have played a part in it, too. Dad said he could remember helicopters spraying it, and to cool off, they would run through it like it was a water sprinkler. No one told them that it was dangerous. He went through all of the problems associated with liver disease until he finally received a transplant. He just had his twenty-year transplant reunion this year. My mom taught me about commitment and compassion by standing by his side the whole time.

I thought about my parents' strength through adversity when I was diagnosed with stage IV colon cancer on September 17, 1998. I was thirty-one, and my daughters were eight and eleven.

For a couple of years, my husband Ronnie and I kept trying to have a baby, but I couldn't get pregnant. I had been extremely fatigued and learned I had anemia. The doctor told us, "You're young; you have two kids and the stress of trying to get pregnant. Just relax a little bit, things will be okay."

By February of 1998, I got to the point where I couldn't breathe or put a couple of words together. Ronnie took me to the emergency room. They ruled out pneumonia, but thought I had some kind of a lung condition. My primary doctor sent me to see a cardiologist. I couldn't get an appointment for several months. They didn't seem very urgent about it, but I was terrified.

After calling throughout the day, we found Dr. Carlos Velasco, who agreed to see me right away. I went through a series of tests until they determined I had a pulmonary embolism. He told us, "Young, healthy females don't have pulmonary embolisms. I think you need to start looking for an underlying cause. With the anemia and other problems you're having, I think you should have a colonoscopy."

My insurance wouldn't pay for a colonoscopy, so they just treated me for the pulmonary embolism. He later told me I was one of three patients he had treated (at that time) who survived a pulmonary embolism. A couple of weeks later, I had a sigmoidoscopy, which was clean.

We went back to normal life, just thinking my problem was one of those things nobody could explain.

In September, I had a blockage they assumed arose from scar tissue from my C-sections years ago. The doctors blamed the adhesions for all my problems, so I went into surgery to clean them up.

That's how they found the colon cancer and three spots on my liver. The doctor said, "You have about six months to live. Go home and get your affairs in order. There's one treatment available for colon cancer; it's been around forever. You've got very advanced cancer, so it's not going to help you."

We literally went from planning a baby to planning a funeral. Ronnie and I put a big red X on the calendar to mark the date and started talking about what we wanted to do with those six months. We put our house up for sale, sold it immediately, and moved to the country.

I was trying to figure out how to tell our kids—not only why we were moving, but what was going to be changing for them. I found the ACOR listserv (ACOR.org) and asked how to prepare my children for life without me. A gentleman named Shelly Weiler, who also had stage IV colon cancer, wrote me back and said, "I have a daughter your age and I would not let her give up out of pride; you shouldn't give up either." He sent me a list of oncologists in Texas and encouraged me to start treatment. Because of him, I started 5-FU, which was and still is the mainstay for colon cancer treatment.

Over the next few months, Shelly and I wrote back and forth. He always encouraged me and was a light in the darkness for me. I didn't realize how sick he was; he passed away about six months after we met. When he died, I remember sitting on my back porch and crying because this person who had helped me and who was encouraging me to live was no longer there.

They didn't do scans back then like they do now, and I didn't under-stand what I do now. I just knew it was bad and that the doctors told me I was going to die. You're supposed to follow the doctor's orders, right? People will tell you when I moved there, all I talked about was I was dying. The first year, I had three friends who took me out to lunch or shopping in between treatments. They threw me a birthday party and bought me very lavish presents, thinking I wouldn't be here the next. You know, they're still buying birthday presents for me fifteen years later!

For the first five years we started living, but the dying was always in the back of our minds. Everything we did was shadowed by the fact that I was going to die. We made every experience like it was going to be our last—the camping trip, the fishing trip. I don't think the girls realized we were thinking in that direction until much later.

I went on several different treatments, including a clinical trial with 5-FU, and interleukin 2, and then a combination of 5-FU, leucovorin, and irinotecan. Even though I started getting scanned regularly, I didn't know how many tumors I had or where they were located. We just followed everything the doctors said. I wasn't a self-advocate at all. I think ignorance was bliss back then, because I knew they expected me to die.

Before cancer, I was very happy being a housewife and taking care of my kids. I didn't worry about having a lot of friends or meeting new people. Cancer, in many ways, opened up my life to a whole new world. I started to go to a cancer support group where I met fellow CancerCare social worker Keith Lyons. I could call him and talk about my fears. I had an outlet for my pity parties with Keith and other friends I met through Association of Cancer Online Resources (ACOR.org) and Colon Cancer Alliance. We were sharing experiences, and I learned from them about managing side effects and new treatments.

In 2004, I had two lung lesions, and about 70 percent of my liver had tumors in it. The doctor told me there wasn't anything else he could do. I was very fatigued and my color was getting bad, but I was still functioning just because I didn't know what else to do. My memory was failing, and I started acting strange. For instance, I have no memory of a trip we took to Arkansas. The kids told me later if something was missing, they looked in the freezer because I put everything there. I look back now and I realize I was on the verge of liver failure.

The Colon Cancer Alliance offered me a scholarship to come to their conference around this time. I was good friends with the group's president, who told me, "We're going to have some pretty good surgeons here. Bring your scans, let them look at them, and maybe they can give you some ideas of what you can do."

I went to the conference and was excited to meet all of the people I'd been talking to on the phone and through letters. I think I cried the whole two days; it was so wonderful. The last night we were there, the surgeon looked at my scans as me and my friends were standing around. I guess everybody expected him to say something hopeful or inspiring. The surgeon looked up at Ronnie and said, "There's not anybody who can help your wife; she's dying." We left the conference knowing we were coming home to hospice.

Before we made the decision, we went to my oncologist, who confirmed what the surgeon said. We came home and had a family meeting to tell the kids and my parents. I sent an email telling all my buddies we chose hospice and there just wasn't anything left for me.

A fellow stage IV colon cancer survivor and friend of mine and a brilliant guy, Gordon Gwosdow, wrote back to me about Sir Spheres, a targeted radiation procedure in which they inject millions of radioactive Y-90-filled microspheres directly to liver tumors. He told me, "My doctor, Jim Thomas, is doing it, and it's a great procedure! It's going to save your life!" He gave me Jim's phone number and told me to call him.

I just didn't want to hear again there wasn't anything they could do. Gordon must have called me twelve times that day, every hour or so, and asked, "Did you call Jim?" I finally called and Dr. Thomas told me, "Send your scan, and I'll see if I think you're a candidate. I'll be honest; it may be too late, but I'll look."

After sending the scans, he told us I was a good candidate and referred me to Dr. Travis VanMeter in Texas. My insurance denied the procedure, but I didn't know then about appealing an insurance claim. Luckily, in January 2005, Ronnie's company insurance changed to Aetna, and they approved it. On January 5, I had my procedure and a few months afterward, my oncologist put me on the oral chemotherapy, Xeloda.

When I was really sick and not sure whether Sir Spheres would help, I remembered a conversation with my friend Keith who told me, "As long as you're alive, you have choices. There's nothing you can do about the way you're going to die. But you have all the power in the world to choose how you're going to live. No matter how bad things get, you have the power to make that moment good or bad."

He sent me a photo with "hope" written in the sand, and said, "Nobody can take your hope away. Whether it's hoping for a peaceful breath, for another minute with your kids, or to squeeze Ronnie's hand, it's there. Whenever you start to doubt, just look at this photo and it'll be right there."

I kept that photo with me wherever I went. Some days, I wouldn't stop looking at it. That was the tipping point for me. We stopped thinking about me dying from cancer and instead started thinking about grabbing each day and living in the present. I wasn't dying from cancer; I was living with cancer.

As Keith told me, "People always think you're either going to die from cancer or you're going to get cured. In your case, you may not ever be able to get rid of it, but think of how you're feeling right now. If you start feeling worse, think of how you're going to get through this challenge and embrace it."

His words helped me shift my perspective. Instead of looking forward, I live moment by moment. It's all about embracing things I can do while I am here.

Three months after my Sir Spheres procedure, they did a scan and the doctor said, "This is incredible! Your tumors have reduced by 30 percent! Everything is looking better than we could have ever imagined!"

Six months out, I had a 65 percent reduction in the tumors. I went from not being able to walk to my mailbox, to being able to walk a mile and a half.

They asked me back to the Colon Cancer Alliance conference, and people all around me were saying, "My gosh, we thought you'd be dead! You don't look like the same person as last year; this is absolutely amazing!"

A friend of mine there, Dusty Weaver, told me, "You've got to go to Capitol Hill and tell your story!" I told him I couldn't get in front of people because I was a shy person, but he kept encouraging me. Finally I agreed to go to training, and from there, my advocacy work began.

I had been volunteering for the Colon Cancer Alliance, coordinating the Buddy Program, which matched people all over the country with fellow colon cancer survivors. In 2006, *The Today Show* producers were doing a segment about Colon Cancer Awareness Month and called the Alliance for people to be on the show. They recommended me and two other members to be on their program. They flew Ronnie and me to New York to be on the show. It was incredible!

Katie Couric had a gala that night, and she asked Ronnie and me and the two other ladies to attend. Oprah Winfrey, Whoopi Goldberg, and Donald Trump were there. Women wore dresses that probably cost more than my house, and we were in suits I bought from Goodwill. She raised three million dollars in that two-hour dinner.

I had been to only one advocacy training when I was asked to help with reimbursement issues for brachytherapy. They were having problems with radioembolization reimbursement and asked if I would go to DC to talk to Congress about my experience. I had never spent one night, other than hospital stays, away from Ronnie. I was terrified. Ronnie called our contact at Sirtex (the maker of Sir Spheres), Desiree, telling her, "She can go and do this, but you better take care of her."

After she brought me to the hotel, I slept with the hotel phone under my pillow and a chair propped by the door. The next morning, I gathered my courage and walked outside of the hotel room to get coffee. Desiree, in the meantime, called my room to see if I wanted to go to breakfast and couldn't get a hold of me. She had the whole security team looking for me! I did go to the Capitol that day, though, to tell my story. I give Desiree credit for getting me into advocacy work because she really helped me find a voice and to share my story.

That year I was chosen as a delegate for the LIVESTRONG Summit. A few of the speakers talked about how knowledge is power and the importance of being on top of your healthcare. I didn't know the importance of getting my lab results. That really empowered me to start learning more about my own condition, where my tumors were located, and what treatments and clinical trials were available.

One of the speakers talked about coming up with a personal action plan and how you can take your experience and really make a big impact. That was another big turning point for me. A couple of months later, I started laying the groundwork for YES Beat Liver Tumors, an organization which provides information, resources, support, and hope to people affected by liver cancer.

The first year, we probably had five hundred dollars. Since then we have grown and grown. We do twelve liver seminars each year, which bring doctors and patients together to build awareness of available treatments and procedures. I have a conference in New York next week and one in Dallas this weekend. I literally could be somewhere almost every day of the week, but then I wouldn't have a life. I'm trying to cut back on my travel and let other people help with the seminars.

I love traveling and being busy, though. I get tired, but it's a different kind of tired when I stop and I'm not traveling. When I stop, I have time to think about my feet hurting from neuropathy. The more I go, the less I worry about what's happening physically. I think, *Cancer, catch me if you can.*

We have stopped worrying so much about getting rid of all the cancer, but instead just how can we buy more time. After the Sir Spheres, I started becoming much more in tune with what treatments were available. I call it hitchhiking—when one treatment stops working, we go to another.

My last scan showed I had a little bit of growth in a lung tumor. We had several options and had to decide "which car to get into." We chose a targeted procedure called radiofrequency (RFA) ablation. I've had two other RFAs, one lung and one liver RFA in the past, so this will probably be the last time I can do a lung RFA. I have also had CyberKnife.

There are two more colon cancer drugs that were approved last year that are options for me. I'm looking at promising clinical trials, which I think are going to be breakthroughs in the next year or two.

I don't always hitchhike to a new treatment; sometimes I choose treatments I've been on previously. I have been on my last chemo (Oxaliplatin and Xeloda) about four times. When we make choices, we'll say, "I hitched a ride with this car before, but it's okay because it was a good ride." We hope it works as well as it did before.

I balance all of this by focusing on each moment and living every minute to the fullest. If I get lost on thinking about how I'm going to die, I will be lost in fear and stress. A very dear friend of mine said when she was in hospice, "I'm not afraid to die; I just don't want to." I think that wraps it up for me, too.

I think about all of the people that I have met, and how they've shaped my life. If it weren't for Shelly Weiler, I probably would have died without chemo. I met another friend, Jean, ten years ago when she was diagnosed with stage IV liver cancer. She was crying, scared, and had no one to talk to who understood. We were both young and with the same cancer, and I was glad to support her. Once Jean got through her surgery and was doing well, she started supporting me. She sent me a little rock with a bumble-bee on it with a note that said, "A bumblebee's not supposed to be able to fly; you're not supposed to survive. But the bumblebee flies and you're going to survive."

Kevin Lebret-White, my mentor from Imerman Angels, who recently passed away, also made a huge impact on my life. For the last eight years, he and I fought this battle together. We climbed a mountain together, and high-fived at the top. We marched the halls of Congress together and wrote "HOPE" on the Capitol sand.

Each and every one of us plays a part in helping the other; it's just a continuum of sharing and caring. And we all share hope with each other. As Keith said, "Your hope may change, and it may not be what it was yesterday or what it will be tomorrow, but you've always got it. Never let anyone take it away."

Lessons Learned

- Find someone else who's been in your shoes. Don't try to do it alone.
- Keep hope alive. Hope moves me forward. It's like a magic wand that transforms the way I live.
- Remember you have choices, not just with cancer treatments, but with how you live.

For more information about Suzanne's organization, Beat Liver Tumors, visit www.beatlivertumors.org.

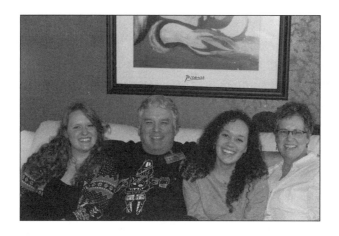

Self-Care Is Job Number One

TERRI DILTS
Seattle, WA
Age 52
Living with stage IV, estrogen/progesterone-, and HER2-positive breast cancer since 2005

I had a tumultuous relationship with my parents. When I was seventeen and a senior in high school, they assigned me over to the courts, deeming me incorrigible. I left the house and lived with a friend's family. I haven't spoken with them since. My mother just never really liked me, and I'm not sure why. I think there was some mental illness there. My father stood by his wife.

I was angry for a while and spent a lot of time self-loathing and self-medicating with drugs and alcohol. I had to learn how to be financially and emotionally responsible for myself. Anger can become poisonous, so at some point I needed to let it go. By doing that, I eventually learned to love myself.

I got married at thirty, and had my first child, Sarah, at thirty-one. I was ready for the adventure, but never anticipated how much she captured my heart. I remember confessing to my husband in the early weeks after she was newborn that I loved her more than him. He wasn't offended at all.

It was important to me to not be like my mother. I was blessed to be able to be a stay-at-home mom until my kids went to school. I think I gave my kids a very strong, centered start in life. That gave me great solace after being diagnosed with cancer.

In August 2000, Katie was getting ready to start full-day kindergarten. Sarah was eight years old. One Saturday morning, I did a breast self-exam in the shower, which I did sporadically. I thought, *What the heck is this? Is this a lump?* I have large, dense breasts so I questioned whether it was a lump or not. I asked my husband to feel my left breast to see if he thought it was lump. He couldn't tell, but he urged me to call the doctor.

Biopsy results showed I had stage IIB breast cancer because of its significant size. They did a sentinel node biopsy, which showed no lymph node involvement. When I heard the word "cancer," I thought, *I'm going to die, and my kids are too young. Can my husband do this without me?*

After I had more time to mull it over, I realized I had no control over this. I thought, *If I am to die, I've given them the best start I could.*

I opted for a lumpectomy with a breast reduction on the other side, which I requested to be done at the same time. After I recovered, we started four rounds of Adriamycin and high dose Cytoxan, followed with two rounds of Taxotere. Once I was done, I did breast radiation and started Tamoxifen. I was estrogen- and progesterone- (ER/PR) and HER2-positive. But Herceptin in 2000 was still experimental, and I didn't qualify for the trial.

So I went on my merry way. I was a survivor; I had the pink T-shirts, hats, and ribbons. I took a part-time job when Katie started kindergarten. I worked throughout my treatment and continued to love my job.

In 2003, I started to have some back pain. I had disc issues after I had Sarah. I didn't associate it with cancer at all because I was unaware of what metastatic meant. After all, my lymph nodes weren't involved. Eventually, I was in so much pain, I was hobbling with a cane. I saw my oncologist every six months and went to an acupuncturist and chiropractor, but none of them suggested a scan.

In December 2005, a friend of a friend who had successful back surgery with some disc problems referred me to a surgeon. I arranged an appointment with the surgeon and had an MRI before I went to see him. He called me after seeing the MRI results and said, "I can't help you; you have tumors in your spine." I was floored!

The next morning my husband and I went to my oncologist. It was hard to focus on all the information he was giving me. I remember he said I had probably four years until something new came down the line that would help me. All I heard was, "You have four years to live." My husband pulled me back to reality emphasizing "until something new came down the line."

My oncologist immediately stopped the Tamoxifen and put me in menopause with Lupron injections and Femara for the ER/PR side of things, and Herceptin, since I was also HER2-positive. I started radiation on the spine to alleviate pain and an older bisphosphonate to strengthen the bones. After radiation, I started low-dose chemotherapy.

I had to pull myself back together because my kids were nine and twelve, and I had to explain this to them without scaring them. My older daughter was a little more aware and concerned. I heard that my younger daughter thought my cancer came back because I had a party to celebrate my five-year mark. You know how kids' minds work. Some adults are like that, too; they're very superstitious.

We were always up-front and honest about cancer in terms they could understand, tempered with "Mom's fighting." We didn't hide anything, but we tried not to burden them with anything either. We did our best not to let it extremely impact their lives. I continued to take them to the school bus and picked them up after. They saw me bald and moving a little slower, but dinner always came. We always made it to the parent-teacher conferences and rewarded them for their good grades. My friend Gayle put together a Share the Care Team, organizing meals and rides for the kids, as needed.

I started gaining strength and learning more about metastatic disease. Everything I read on the Internet said I should be dead. Luckily, I found a local metastatic cancer support group, which was such a ray of hope for me. I saw women who were surviving with metastatic disease fifteen to eighteen years after diagnosis. It was such an eye opener for me and instrumental in changing my mindset to one of hope.

As I researched my disease, I decided I needed to add naturopathic approaches to help manage it. I talked to my oncologist about vitamin C infusions, and he said it was quackery. I wasn't going to convince him or vice versa, so we parted ways. I went to the Seattle Cancer Treatment and Wellness Center because they integrated traditional and complementary treatments. They added vitamin C and a whole bunch of supplements to my treatments, along with a cancer-fighting diet plan.

I did some research and switched to mostly organic foods and eliminated red meat. That was where I started. A lot of the diets I read about seemed too restrictive to me, but now I'm trying to incorporate more changes. I'm reading a couple of books, one by a breast cancer survivor, Elaine Cantin, who recommends eliminating all glucose and adding good fats, such as olive and coconut oils and avocados. Cancer cells need glucose, so the theory is to starve your cancer cells.

I eat a lot of macadamia nuts and salmon, which I love anyway, and use almond flour to bake some low-carb goodies. I avoid all artificial sugars, but stevia is a natural one, so I can use that. I gained forty pounds because of my hormone treatment, but I've since lost twenty-five pounds because I was working on it. There is a fine line between doing the best I can to starve cancer cells and living life to its fullest. If I'm going out to eat with friends and family, I'm going to enjoy a glass of wine. If I stick to my diet 80 percent of the time, I think I'll be doing well.

I went on disability about six months after I ended chemotherapy the second time, which has allowed me to spend a lot of time on self-care. I can nap, meditate, and go to the clinic twice a week for infusions. I'm very conscious of exercising my heart because I was on Adriamycin and now on Herceptin and Perjeta, which are possibly cardio-toxic. I try to do aerobics two to three times a week, along with weight-bearing exercises to keep my bones healthy and strong. I'm doing everything I can to live the best life I can. That's my job now.

My scans have been relatively stable. They showed a significant decrease last year, but my last scan showed a minimal amount of growth. I still do vitamin C infusions, Herceptin, and Perjeta and have switched to Faselodex injections and Armidex for my hormone treatments.

When you look fine in the metastatic world, it's almost a double-edged sword. People will say, "Oh, you look wonderful!" I'll respond, "I wear my cancer well." It doesn't mean everything on the inside is terrific. I have to remind people I'm dealing with a terminal disease, and it's a daily task for me.

My husband is a rock, but sometimes he kind of gets a little lacka-daisical since I've been stable and doing well for a long time. Every once in a while, I remind him, "Just pretend I'm sick." I know it affects him, but not like it affects me.

I can't imagine being the caregiver. It's a difficult role, and I have empathy for each and every one of them. They can let the stresses of work creep in, and cancer shuffles to the back burner. It's a coping method for them.

That's why I think it's important for cancer survivors to be there for each other. I started one of the support groups I now attend because I saw a need for it. Occasionally I'll give a speech about my journey. I enjoy that I can give anybody hope. People come up to me after I've given a speech and say they're inspired and share their story with me, as well.

I volunteer to drive senior citizens to their medical appointments, which is not cancer-related directly, but just giving back to the community. I would feel so abandoned if I didn't have a car and was stuck at home. I only give one or two days a week, but it's been really rewarding.

We're entering an "empty nest" phase of our lives, so I'm trying to find my way. I'm enjoying some art classes and finding a way to be creative. Tonight I have a fused glass class and we're going to make jewelry. It's very exciting for me.

I feel grateful I was able to turn away from self-destructive behavior and emotions from my youth. Cancer has taught me to make self-love and self-care a priority. I believe that and the support of my family, friends, and fellow survivors are the reasons I'm still here. I'm not just living, but living well.

Lessons Learned

- Keep your diagnosis in perspective. There are people living with debilitating diseases like Alzheimer's and Lou Gehrig disease (ALS). Not to diminish what it's like to have stage IV cancer, but knowing there are other people living with diseases helps me alleviate some of my self-pity.
- Keep hope close to your heart. Every time a new treatment comes down the pipeline, I'm full of hope I can extend my life, and my daughters won't have to deal with breast cancer in the future.
- Take care of yourself. By making self-care your first priority, you can extend and improve your quality of life.

Cancer-Related Resources

Many of the following organizations were noted by people who shared their stories in this and my previous book—either because they started them or found them personally helpful.

Aim@Melanoma

3217 Bob O Link Ct.

Plano, TX 75093

www.aimatmelanoma.org

This organization's goal is to increase support for melanoma research, promote prevention and education among the public and medical professionals, and provide resources for patients, survivors, and caregivers.

American Cancer Society

PO Box 22718

Oklahoma City, OK 73123-1718

1-800-ACS-2345 (or 1-866-228-4327 for TTY)

www.cancer.org

The American Cancer Society (ACS) is committed to fighting cancer through balanced programs of research, education, patient service, advocacy, and rehabilitation.

American Institute for Cancer Research

1759 R Street NW

Washington, DC 20009

1-800-843-8114

(DC: 202-328-7744)

www.aicr.org

AICR helps people make choices that reduce their chances of developing cancer, including diet and exercise.

American Lung Association

55 W. Wacker Dr., Ste. 1150
Chicago, IL 60601
Toll Free: 1-800-LUNGUSA
312-801-7630
www.lung.org
The American Lung Association's mission is to save lives by improving
lung health and preventing lung disease.

American Red Cross

2025 E. Street, NW
Washington, DC 20006
Toll Free: 1-800-RED-CROSS (733-2767)
Public Inquiries: 202-303-4498
www.redcross.org
ACR is the leading provider of health and safety courses around the
world. Many local chapters offer courses.

The Annie Appleseed Project

7319 Serrano Terrace
Delray Beach, FL 33446-2215
561-749-0084
annieappleseedpr@aol.com
www.annieappleseedproject.org
The Annie Appleseed Project explores evidence-based, integrative
treatments and methods through its web site and conferences.

Association of Cancer Online Resources (ACOR)

173 Duane St., Ste. 3A
New York, NY 10013-3334
212-226-5525

feedback@acor.org
www.ACOR.org
A collection of online communities designed to provide timely and accurate cancer information.

Be the Match Registry National Marrow Donor Program

www.bethematch.org
Be the Match helps patients afford transplants, find a matching donor, and build a future while it advances medical research.

Beat Liver Tumors (YES)

791 Arnold Paul
Canton, TX 75103
TF Survivor Line 1-877-937-7478
www.beatlivertumors.org
Beat Liver Tumors provides education and information on treatments, and resources such as insurance assistance for people affected by liver tumors (either primary or metastatic).

Breast Cancer Trials.org

3450 California St.
San Francisco, CA 94118
415-476-5777
help-desk@bctrials.org
www.bctrials.org
Trial Alert Service is an easy way to learn about newly listed trials to match your situation.

Breast Friends

14050 SW Pacific Highway, Ste. 201
Tigard, OR 97224
Toll Free: 1-888-386-8048
sharon@breastfriends.org
www.breastfriends.org
Breast Friends is dedicated to improving the quality of life for female cancer patients. It also teaches friends and family specific ways to offer support and appropriate help to the patient.

Camp Kesem

PO Box 452
Culver City, CA 90232
info@campkesem.org
260-225-3736 / 260-22-KESEM
www.campkesem.org
Camp Kesem empowers college student leaders nationwide to create free, life-changing summer camps for children affected by a parent's cancer.

Cancer has Cancer

214-586-0782
contact@cancerhascancer.org
www.cancerhascancer.org
Founded by Heather Rodriguez, who is featured in this book, Cancer has Cancer Group Connect is a worldwide, unique online support group for all types of cancers. Pinche Cancer works with the Hispanic community, where cancer is the number one cause of death. Offers support and information in Spanish.

Cancer Protocol.com

www.cancerprotocol.com
Cancer Protocol.com features peer-reviewed, published studies by well-known academic centers or research institutions.

Cancer Support Community (formerly The Wellness Community/Gilda's Club)

1050 17th St., NW, Ste. 500
Washington, DC 20036
Toll Free: 1-888-793-WELL (9355)
202-659-9709
www.cancersupportcommunity.org
Cancer Support Community provides professional programs of emotional support, education, and hope for people affected by cancer at no charge, so that no one faces cancer alone.

Center for Attitudinal Healing

33 Buchanan Dr.
Dr. Sausalito, CA 94965
415-331-6161
www.healingcenter.org
The Center for Attitudinal Healing integrates practical and spiritual principles into a psychological format to make a choice to experience peace of mind, even in the face of real difficulty.

Children's Brain Tumor Foundation

274 Madison Ave., Ste. 1004
New York, NY 10016
Toll Free: 1-866-228-4673
www.cbtf.org
The Children's Brain Tumor Foundation mission is to improve the treatment, quality of life, and long-term outlook for children with brain and spinal cord tumors.

ClinicalTrials.gov

US National Institutes of Health

Registry and results database of publicly and privately supported clinical studies from around the world.

Colon Cancer Alliance

1025 Vermont Ave., NW, Ste. 1066

Washington, DC 20005

Toll Free: 1-877-422-2030

202-628-0123

www.ccalliance.org

The Colon Cancer Alliance's mission is to knock colon cancer out of the top three cancer killers. The Buddy Program connects new patients and caregivers with a Buddy who has been through the cancer journey before. The Blue Note Fund gives one-time grants to colon cancer patients in active treatment. The organization also offers a clinical trial matching service.

CureSearch for Children's Cancer

4600 East-West Highway, Ste. 600

Bethesda, MD 20814

Toll Free: 1-800-458-6223

info@curesearch.org

www.curesearch.org

CureSearch is a national non-profit foundation that accelerates the cure for children's cancer.

Cutaneous Lymphoma Foundation

PO Box 374

Birmingham, MI 48012

248-644-9014

info@clfoundation.org

www.clfoundation.org

The CL Foundation is dedicated to supporting every person with cutaneous lymphoma by promoting awareness and education, advancing patient care, and facilitating research.

The Few, The Proud, The Forgotten: Camp Lejeune Toxic Water incident information

tftptf@aol.com

www.tftptf.com

A website with information for those exposed to long-term chemical release into drinking water near Camp Lejeune from 1957–1987.

GregsMission.org

Founded by Greg Cantwell, who is featured in this book, Greg's Mission supports patients, family members, and caregivers of those with brain cancer.

Imerman Angels

205 W. Randolph, 19th floor

Chicago, IL 60606

312-274-5529

Toll Free: 1-877-274-5529

info@imermanangels.org

www.imermanangels.org

Founded by cancer survivor Jonny Imerman, the organization partners a person fighting cancer with someone who has beaten the same type of cancer.

Inflammatory Breast Cancer (IBC) Research Foundation

PO Box 2805

Lafayette, IN 47996

Toll Free: 1-877-786-7422

information@mail.ibcresearch.org
www.ibcresearch.org
IBC Research Foundation focuses on research and awareness of
inflammatory breast cancer.

The Leukemia and Lymphoma Society National Office
1311 Mamaroneck Ave., Ste. 310
White Plains, NY 10605
Toll Free: 1-888-557-7177
914-949-5213
www.lls.org
Helps blood cancer patients live better, longer lives and offers support
and information for patients and their families and caregivers.

LIVESTRONG
2201 E. Sixth St.
Austin, TX 78702
1-877-236-8820
For Cancer Support: 855-220-7777
www.livestrong.org
LIVESTRONG unites people to fight cancer and pursue an agenda
focused on prevention, access to screening and care, improvement of
the quality of life for survivors, and investment in research.

Living Beyond Breast Cancer
354 West Lancaster Ave., Ste. 224
Haverford, PA 19041
Toll Free: 1-855-807-6386
610-645-4567
mail@lbbc.org
www.lbbc.org
A national education and support organization dedicated to improving
survivors' quality of life and helping them take an active role in their
ongoing recovery or management of cancer.

Lung Cancer Alliance

888 16th St. NW, Ste. 150
Washington, DC 20006
202-463-2080
Lung Cancer Information Line: 1-800-298-2436 (9 a.m. to 5 p.m. Eastern Time)
info@lungcanceralliance.org
www.lungcanceralliance.org
The Lung Cancer Alliance is the only national non-profit organization dedicated solely to patient support and advocacy for people living with lung cancer and those at risk for the disease.

Make-A-Wish Foundation

4742 N. 24th St., Ste. 400
Phoenix, AZ 85016
Toll Free 1-800-722-9474
602-279-9474
www.wish.org
Make-A-Wish grants the wish of a child diagnosed with a life-threatening medical condition, believing that a wish experience can be a game-changer for the child and his loved ones.

Metastatic Breast Cancer Network

PO Box 1449
New York, NY 10159
Toll Free: 1-888-500-0370
mbcn@mbcn.org
www.mbcn.org
A national, independent, non-profit, all volunteer, patient-led organization for those with metastatic breast cancer.

Miracle Party Foundation

17061 E. Eldorado Circle
Aurora, CO 80013
720-295-1613
www.miraclepartyfoundation.org
The foundation hosts an annual "Miracle Party" in the Denver area for childhood cancer patients and their families from all over the US.

National Breast Cancer Coalition

1101 17th St., NW, Ste. 1300
Washington, DC 20036
Toll Free: 1-800-622-2838
202-296-7477
www.breastcancerdeadline2020.org
NBBC's mission is to know how to end breast cancer by January 1, 2020.

National Cancer Institute

BG 9609 MSC 9760
9609 Medical Center Dr.
Bethesda, MD 20892-9760
1-800-4-CANCER (1-800-422-6237)
Monday to Friday, 8 a.m. to 8 p.m., English and Spanish
www.cancer.gov
The National Cancer Institute coordinates the National Cancer Program, which conducts and supports research, training, health information dissemination, and other programs. Its focus is on the cause, diagnosis, prevention, treatment, rehabilitation of cancer, and the continuing care of cancer patients and their families.

NCI also includes the Physician Data Query, its comprehensive cancer database. It contains summaries on a wide range of cancer topics, including a registry of 8,000+ open and 19,000+ closed cancer clinical trials from around the world.

Pancreatic Cancer Action Network

1500 Rosecrans Ave., Ste. 200
Manhattan Beach, CA 90266
Toll Free: 1-877-272-6226
310-725-0025
email@pancan.org
www.pancan.org
PCAN is a non-profit organization which focuses on advocacy, awareness, and support for cancer of the pancreas with local chapters throughout the US.

Patient Advocate Foundation (PAF)

421 Butter Farm Rd.
Hampton, VA 23666
Toll Free: 1-800-532-5274
help@patientadvocate.org
www.patientadvocate.org
PAF's Patient Services provides patients with arbitration, mediation, and negotiation to settle issues with access to care, medical debt, and more.

Susan G. Komen for the Cure

5005 LBJ Freeway, Suite 250
Dallas, TX 75244
1-877 GO KOMEN (1-877-465-6636)
www.komen.org
The world's largest grassroots network of breast cancer survivors and activists, working to save lives, empower people, ensure quality care for all, and energize science to find the cures for breast cancer.

The Ulman Cancer Fund for Young Adults

6310 Stevens Forest Rd., Ste. 210
Columbia, MD 21046
Hours: Monday–Friday, 9 a.m.–5 p.m.
(unless scheduling a meeting, please call before stopping by as we have a small office)
410-964-0202, ext. 107
Toll Free: 1-888-393-FUND (3863)
info@ulmanfund.org
www.ulmanfund.org
Founded by Doug Ulman, now CEO and president of the Lance Armstrong Foundation, The Ulman Fund enhances lives by supporting, educating, and connecting young adults affected by cancer and their loved ones.

Young Survival Coalition

80 Broad St., Ste. 1700
New York, NY 10004
Toll Free: 1-877-972-1011
www.youngsurvival.org
YSC works with survivors, caregivers, and the medical, research, advocacy, and legislative communities to increase the quality and quantity of life for women diagnosed with breast cancer ages forty and under.

CALIFORNIA
Breast Cancer Angels

6889 Andrew Way
Cypress, CA 90630
714-898-8900
www.breastcancerangels.org
Breast Cancer Angels provides financial and emotional assistance for women and families in certain areas of California as they are going through breast cancer treatment.

MASSACHUSETTS

The Ellie Fund

475 Hillside Ave.
Needham, MA 02494
781-449-0100
info@elliefund.org
www.elliefund.org
The Ellie Fund improves the health and welfare of women and families undergoing breast cancer treatment in Massachusetts. Its free services include transportation to medical appointments, childcare, housekeeping, groceries, and nutritious meals.

Hope in Bloom

202 Bussey St.
Dedham, MA 02026
781-381-3597
info@hopeinbloom.org
www.hopeinbloom.org
Hope in Bloom plants gardens free of charge at the homes of women and men undergoing treatment for breast cancer. The program operates throughout Massachusetts.

OHIO

Cincinnati Dreams Come True

PO Box 42890
Cincinnati, OH 45242-0890
513-891-1941
www.cincinnatidreams.org
Cincinnati Dreams Come True serves children under the age of eighteen who live within a hundred-mile radius of Cincinnati, or who are regular patients of Cincinnati Children's Hospital Medical Center.

Pink Ribbon Girls

PO Box 58420
Cincinnati, OH 45258
937-545-6199
info@pinkribbongirls.org
www.pinkribbongirls.org
Pink Ribbon Girls provides support and services, such as free house-keeping, meals, transportation, and childcare for southwest Ohio survivors going through cancer treatment. They also have national online community that provides support and education to young breast cancer survivors.

TEXAS

CanCare

9575 Katy Freeway, Suite 428
Houston, Texas 77024
Toll Free: 1-888-461-0028
713-461-0028
www.cancare.org
CanCare provides emotional support to those currently facing a battle with cancer.